The discoverer of pantothenic acid, an important member of the vitamin B family, Dr. Roger J. Williams also concentrated and christened folic acid, another B vitamin, in his pioneering studies of vitamins and nutrition. At the Clayton Foundation Biochemical Institute of the University of Texas at Austin, during his Directorship (1941-1963), more vitamins and their variants were discovered than in any other laboratory in the world. The first biochemist to be elected president of the American Chemical Society, Dr. Williams was a member of the National Academy of Sciences and the recipient of numerous awards and degrees. *The Wonderful World Within You* is an important step toward improving nutrition for everyone—young and old.

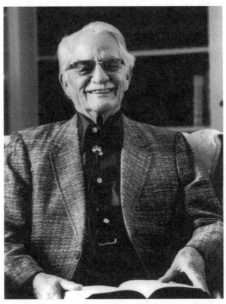

Roger J. Williams, 1893-1988

SELECTED BOOKS
BY ROGER J. WILLIAMS

Free and Unequal, 1953
Biochemical Individuality, 1956
Alcoholism: The Nutritional Approach, 1959
Nutrition In A Nutshell, 1962
You Are Extraordinary, 1967
*Nutrition Against Disease: Environmental
    Prevention*, 1971
Physicians' Handbook of Nutritional Science, 1975
The Wonderful World Within You, 1977
The Prevention of Alcoholism Through Nutrition, 1982
The Advancement of Nutrition, 1982
*Rethinking Education: The Coming Age of
    Enlightenment*, 1986

For more information about Williams' books, articles, and background, visit the Internet Website devoted to his work: http://www.cm.utexas.edu/faculty/williams.

THE WONDERFUL WORLD WITHIN YOU:
Your Inner Nutritional Environment

DR. ROGER J. WILLIAMS

THE WONDERFUL WORLD WITHIN YOU:
YOUR INNER NUTRITIONAL ENVIRONMENT
Bio-Communications Press / April 1998

BIO-COMMUNICATIONS PRESS
3100 North Hillside Avenue
Wichita, Kansas 67219 USA

ISBN 0-942333-12-8
Previously published by Bantam Books, Inc., ISBN 0-553-10411-X
Library of Congress Catalog Card Number: 87-70770

Revised Edition

Published in The United States of America

BCP and Bio-Communications Press are service marks of The Center
for the Improvement of Human Functioning International, Inc.

CONTENTS

PREFACE TO 1998 EDITION

I am pleased to introduce this updated edition of a wonderful book whose birth I watched and assisted. Its gestation began about 1975, soon after I joined the author's research group here at the University of Texas. I marveled at professor Williams' amazing ability—in his early eighties—to appear each morning with drafts of new sections, beautifully written in simple, clear words. I savored, as I think you will, his broad knowledge, his philosophical spirit, and his enthusiastic, yet scientific, vision for the advancement of nutrition. And I was struck by how much each of us may differ from the mythical "average person"—in our physical bodies, in our biochemistry and nutrition, and in our minds and abilities. Williams helps us appreciate the truly wonderful world within ourselves and within others.

Of course, much has happened since this book was born in 1977—and since Williams died in 1988, at age 94. Most excitingly, we now recognize a new nutrient—a new "growth and maintenance chemical," as Williams calls them here. It is alpha-linolenic acid, an omega-3 fatty acid. It is nearly the same as (but very different from) linoleic acid, which was first recognized as a nutrient about 50 years earlier. Alpha-linolenic acid, and substances we make from it, play crucial roles in our brains, eyes, blood and most other tissues. It shines new light on the prevention and treatment of heart disease, cancer, and many other disorders.

Williams would be excited, too, by recent recognition of protective "phytochemicals" in plant foods. Phytochemicals are not essential like nutrients, but nevertheless they play valuable roles in our bodies. We know of hundreds, and there may be thousands. Many are antioxidants that help prevent cancer and heart disease. Others help us resist infections and maintain normal blood pressure. We are only beginning to understand them. Phytochemicals occur in all whole plant foods—vegetables, fruits, nuts, whole grains, beans, teas, herbs, and seaweed. They add new importance to the message in this book and elsewhere that we focus our diets on whole foods, instead of the added sugars, added fats, and refined grains that dominate most Western diets.

Another notable advance since 1977 is growing evidence that Williams was (and still is) ahead of the pack regarding heart disease: Atherosclerosis "is a complex problem that is not solved merely by eating less fat or avoiding cholesterol-containing foods . . . . there is much to be said for the idea that if we eat the right foods and get the right assortment of growth and maintenance chemicals, cholesterol and cholesterol deposits will take care of themselves" (chapter X). Today there is much more to say for this idea. Although popular opinion still dwells on avoiding cholesterol and fat, most researchers now de-emphasize *dietary* cholesterol, and some de-emphasize *blood* cholesterol. Many are studying diverse nutrients that help prevent the damage that precedes cholesterol deposits, especially damage from homocysteine and oxidized cholesterol. Others study the "paradox" of populations with high fat diets but little heart disease. The spotlight is strongly shifting toward Williams' early focus on those many growth and maintenance chemicals that protect us against heart disease, while they allow naturally-occurring fats and cholesterol to serve the many positive roles that nature intended.

The evolving story of heart disease illustrates one of Williams' gifts. Although he was a pioneer and visionary, he had keen insight, and he stayed firmly rooted in basic principles. He avoided many passing fancies and oversimplifications, some of which still linger. Even after 20 years of scientific progress, his presentation remains fresh and relevant. Besides a few changes related to the recognition of alpha-linolenic acid as a nutrient, revised estimates of nutrient needs (Table 1), and the updates described below, there are few changes in this edition.

The "cartwheel-type" nutrient diagrams for 40 foods (chapter XV) are completely updated for this edition. They now include the newly recognized omega-3-fatty acid nutrients (alpha-linolenic acid and its progeny, EPA and DHA). Also new is the amino acid histidine (whose status is more certain now) and dietary fiber, for which there was too little data in 1977. All nutrient data and food prices used in the diagrams and captions are updated, mostly from U.S. Department of Agriculture reports. The new diagrams are computer-drawn "NutriCircles"—a big relief to me, as I recall many hours spent proofing and correcting the original, artist-drawn diagrams. Although only the original 40 foods are included here, diagrams for over 2000 foods are now available (in color). NutriCircles software for IBM-type personal computers is available from the publisher of this book and from my associates (see pages near the end of this book).

We are fortunate to have this new edition. It neatly summarizes Williams' lifetime of wisdom about many topics: nutrition, wholesome foods, nutritional supplements, our marvelous individual differences, preventing alcoholism, and finding a healthy and satisfying life. What more could we ask of one book?

Donald R. Davis, Ph.D.
Biochemical Institute
The University of Texas at Austin
January 1998

AUTHOR'S PREFACE

Is this book for you?

Developing and maintaining a healthy bodily mechanism is a lifelong endeavor. There is no stage in life at which we can safely neglect the problem of proper maintenance. If you are fifteen years old, you will be interested in the optimal growth and development of your own internal machinery. If you are twenty, growth may be almost complete but development and maintenance are still taking place. If you are thirty, your interest in healthful development will probably have expanded to include your own children. If you are forty or older, the story is the same, with variations. As long as you have life, you can hope for better days, a better life, and better health.

There is unity in life. The boy is the father of the man; the girl is on the road to womanhood. Many of the troubles that arise in middle age are on the way in youth. How one fares in old age may depend on how well one has prepared in youth and middle age. One of the tragedies of middle and old age is failure to recognize that illnesses do not arise out of nothing. People who are visited with sickness late in life often have no idea that they may have been paving the way for it for years.

There is another kind of unity in life. We individuals are not islands; we are bound together in a thousand ways by interdependence and common interests. If you have brothers or sisters, they are part of your life. The bond between husband and wife is strong; bonds between parents and children may be stronger. No one will read this book without thinking of others and of how the insights he or she is gaining might be utilized by those with whom he or she rubs elbows physically, emotionally, or intellectually.

In order to take care of one's complex physical equipment, it is necessary, at least partially, to understand it. There is no simple recipe for living. If one is not willing to learn, he or she must take the consequences. These may include living a life less rich in energy and satisfaction than it might have been.

I have designed this book to help people of all ages to do their living with greater expertise. Those who patiently read what follows will not only learn how to do a better job of living; they will also be convinced that how they care for their internal machinery is not a trifling matter: it can make a world of difference.

No other book I know of presents, or claims to present, similar insights into these problems.

Roger J. Williams

THE WONDERFUL WORLD WITHIN YOU: Your Inner Nutritional Environment

I

WHAT THIS BOOK IS ABOUT

This book is *about you*. Since you know yourself better than anyone else, you must help me make it a book *for you*. Though I hope you will live happily ever after, you will have to write the happy ending for yourself. My wishes will be fulfilled if you greatly increase your knowledge of yourself and apply what you have learned in your lifelong experiment of guiding your own distinctive destiny. You will discover, if you have not already, that you are an extraordinary person with many fine potentialities that can easily remain unrealized.

Sometimes it is said that "you are what you eat." It is literally true that there is nothing in our bodies that is not built from what we eat. All the details of our bodies, even their microscopic and submicroscopic structures, have to be built using materials we put into our mouths as food. Bodies can be well or poorly built simply because of the quality of the food that is eaten.

Like human beings, animals depend on the nutrition they receive for good development, energy, health, alertness, and attractiveness. It is no accident that prize-winning cats and dogs are well nourished and that cattle direct from ordinary pasture feeding are unlikely to win blue ribbons. Because large animals are expensive and inconvenient to work with in laboratories, rats and other small animals are often used for nutritional experimentation. Permit me, therefore, to introduce to you four male rats I have worked with: Peewee, Puny, Norm (for normal), and Super (see figures 1 and 2). Exactly the same age, the four were photographed together on their fifteenth birthday —when they were fifteen weeks old. Throughout their lives Peewee, Puny, Norm, and Super were treated exactly alike in every respect but one. Each rat had in his cage at all times a fresh supply of food and water. Each received nothing but pure wholesome food. Each was given all the food he wanted. The foods selected for the different rats, however, were far from identical.

At the beginning of the experiment, the four weaned baby rats looked alike. If we had given Peewee the same food as Super, he would have been just as well developed as Super at fifteen weeks. If, on the other hand, Super had received the food Peewee got, he would have looked like Peewee. The *quality* of the food was the only factor which could have made a difference in their development. Poor Peewee, no doubt, had the internal urge to be healthy, vigorous, and mature-looking like Super, but he wasn't given a good supply of the materials he needed to build

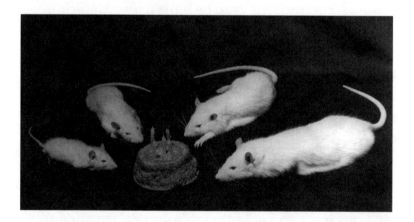

Figure 1. Peewee, Puny, Norm, and Super are at their fifteenth birthday party (fifteen weeks). They are exactly the same age and have been treated alike. Each has been given all the pure, wholesome food he could eat. The only difference is in the nutritional quality of the food selections provided.

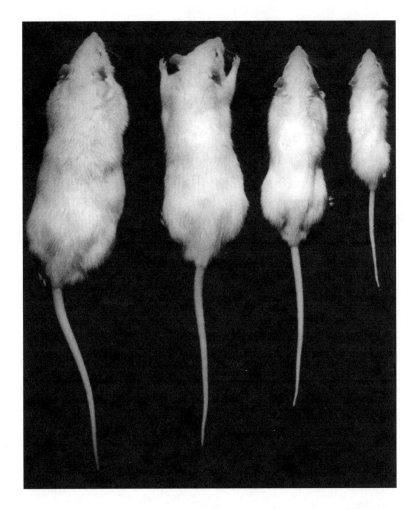

Figure 2. The same four rats are shown side by side, for contrast.

himself. He was like a contractor assigned to build a house without all of the required lumber, nails, cement, bricks, and mortar. Puny and Norm were partially successful in building healthy bodies because they had a partial supply of the nutrients their bodies needed.

Besides Peewee, Puny, Norm, and Super, we raised a few other rats in the same way. To see how their internal organs were affected by the differ-

3

ent levels of nourishment, we painlessly put to sleep one Peewee rat and one Super rat, then dissected out their brains, hearts, kidneys, and testicles for comparison. In figure 3, you can see that in the Peewee rat everything is underdeveloped.

In total body size Peewee was badly stunted. He weighed forty-five grams. The kidneys and heart of the second Peewee rat weighed about one-fourth as much as the corresponding organs of the second Super rat. The second Peewee's testicles weighed only about one-fifteenth as much as the second Super's. By fifteen weeks a rat should be sexually mature. Peewee was much like a boy of six.

It is particularly notable that Peewee's brain weighed about 20 percent less than Super's. The brain is the most important and well-guarded organ in the body. If a mature rat is starved to death, its body loses a large part of its weight, but brain weight at death remains almost unchanged. At weaning, a rat has all the brain cells it will ever have, and at that time the brain is relatively large. From then on, the brain cells merely mature and fill out; the brain grows only a little. Peewee was old enough to be in Rat High School, but his underdeveloped brain would probably not have permitted him to pass the fourth-grade maze.

Rats are engaged largely in finding and eating food, sleeping, reproducing, and avoiding enemies. These activities are greatly influenced by the kind of food consumed day by day. You can easily imagine which of the four would have won if they had been competing for a limited amount of food or an attractive mate, and which would most likely have lost his life if a hungry tomcat had come upon the scene.

Human beings are far more complex than rats. They do what rats can do, and much more. Many things human beings can do are completely out of

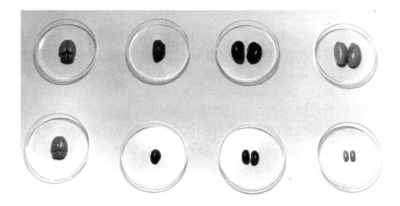

Figure 3. The brain, heart, kidneys, and testicles of a Super-sized rat are shown in the top row. In the bottom row are the corresponding organs of a Peewee-sized rat. The size of these organs (in rats of the same age) is diminished owing to poor quality nutrition.

reach of all beasts. We can read and enjoy literature, ponder about life and the universe, absorb the thoughts of past ages, and develop original ideas. We can appreciate and enjoy art, music, sculpture, and drama. Our agile minds make it possible for us to enjoy playing and watching complex games. Many of us comprehend advanced forms of mathematics and apply them to the solution of problems that would be of no interest to a beast. We can look with seeing eyes at all aspects of the physical, chemical, biological, and aesthetic world around us. We can appreciate and cultivate the moral sense of decency and the beauty of love.

Human nutrition is vastly more interesting than rat nutrition because human nutrition greatly influences all human capabilities. All activities associated with our being human can be performed at higher levels if body and brain development are complete.

Our moral sense prevents us from performing an experiment with human babies comparable to the rat experiment I have described. However, it is easy to find children almost as poorly nourished as Peewee and in no better condition than Puny.

Rats and human beings, because of the enormous gap between them, do not react in precisely the same ways to malnutrition. Malnutrition in young rats is easy to discern. Either they die or their condition is dramatically reflected in their size and weight. Human beings also may die or be stunted by malnutrition; more frighteningly, they can partly lose their unique human powers: the ability to read, think, enjoy literature, art, music, games, mathematics, and nature. Such impairments do not necessarily show on the surface, but the inner life is damaged. A malnourished youngster is underdeveloped mentally and physically and lacks attractiveness, vigor, alertness, ambition, poise, and other valuable human qualities.

Poor quality food is not the only cause of difficulty, of course. Suppose that we had given Peewee, Puny, Norm, and Super excellent diets but at the same time slipped small, graded doses of arsenic or some other poison into the food of all but Super. Too much poison would have killed these three animals just as surely as very poor nutrition can act like a poison. People who would be appalled at the idea of putting arsenic or any other poison into their food may, through ignorance or indifference, be producing similar effects in themselves by choosing their food unwisely.

In later chapters we shall discuss why it is difficult to obtain really excellent nutrition, as well as the meaning and consequences of just "getting by" nutritionally as Peewee, Puny, and Norm did. If you are young, you can probably get by (perhaps to middle age) without devoting much special thought to your own nutrition; but to achieve full development, vigor, health, and a long life, you may have to approach this

6

problem with a good deal of intelligence.

You may now want to ask yourself some questions and begin the search for answers. Suppose a dozen levels of nourishment are available to you. At what level are you now operating? Are you below average, average, above average, or near the top? Would it be worth the required time and effort to try to climb to a higher level?

Before we discuss your nutrition more fully, however, let us think more about *you*, about your place in the scheme of things, and particularly about the marvelous living units within you that make up your body. It is these remarkable living cells that have a crucial need for continuous good nourishment.

II

YOU, ME, AND A PARTNERSHIP

Why am I writing this book? The answer involves you. To achieve certain objectives, I need your cooperation, and I, therefore, propose an active partnership between us.

I will help you make your body mechanisms operate more effectively. You can then help yourself more effectively to attain whatever you want from life. This is a promise. In return, you can help in my campaign to educate people to understand that the quality of the food they consume is vital in determining the quality of their lives—a campaign based upon sound scientific facts and principles. You must learn that it is an exacting task, requiring conscientious head work, to furnish an excellent internal environment to the cells and tissues of your body. When you understand this fully you can do a great deal, quietly and inoffensively, to further the campaign.

If you are a student in high school or college, I am particularly interested in our partnership. You are the kind of person who has most to gain and most potential for bringing about change. You can greatly influence your teachers, your parents, your doctors, your friends, and others. If you are older, you also have much to gain because the influence of good nutrition never ceases to exert itself on your life and health. If you are a parent, you have children to consider; if you are a professional person, you may be in an especially good position to spread the news about how good nutrition can improve the quality of life. Everyone has influence. I want to foster a grass-roots movement to abolish nutritional illiteracy.

Because partnerships are often hazardous, you should be cautious about accepting my offer. I should like to give you enough background about myself to enable you to understand the basis of my promises, to have some confidence in what I have to say, and to feel sure that you are not being sucked into accepting unscientific, faddist notions. You must be convinced that I am an honest scientist with something solid to say—not a charlatan who might unwittingly lead you astray.

Let us begin our discussion by recognizing ourselves for what we are. Everything in the universe can be viewed with different perspectives. We human beings are no exceptions and what we appear to be depends in large part on the viewpoint.

From the outer reaches of our Milky Way our sun would appear as a very tiny speck of light. Yet from our viewpoint it seems in a sense to be the source of all energy and life. Sun worshippers have abounded since before recorded history began.

From outside our solar system our earth would look like a tiny object shining only by reflected light, but from our closer viewpoint it is our still spacious home where we and about four billion other human beings live.

From an airplane the people on earth are tiny specks moving around on the surface like ants on a dung hill. From a closer perspective, however, human beings are marvelous in detail and of unbelievable complexity. In their own way they are more wonderful than anything else we can observe in the universe.

Because you are a human being, you have a body whose structure is both elegant and splendid. It is a highly complicated, dynamic, superbly organized system consisting of something like 60 trillion living specks of different sizes and shapes, called cells: about 600 times as many of them as there are stars in the Milky Way.

Each living cell in your body is magnificent. There is no typical or average cell; different types have distinctive structures, each is marvelous in design and organization. A cell of average size contains about 1 quadrillion specks of different sizes and shapes, called molecules, some hundreds of times as large as others. Unlike cells, the molecules, though often in rapid motion, are not alive. A cell has about 10,000 times as many molecules as the Milky Way has stars.

Thus, in the universe there are specks and specks. Our sun is a speck; our earth is a speck; human beings are specks; body cells are specks; molecules are specks. Atoms within molecules are specks; the electrons, protons, positrons, mesons, etc., within atoms are specks. It all depends upon our perspective. You and I can be proud of being specks, for what marvelous specks we are! What a wonderful speck *you* are, and in your world and the world of humanity *you* are important. All the specks in the universe travel in their respective orbits. You are in the human orbit.

These specks within specks remind me of Augustus De Morgan's rhyme:

Great fleas have little fleas upon their backs
to bite 'em, And little fleas have lesser fleas,
and so *ad infinitum.*

It is high praise to be described as "a person of parts." And that is certainly what you are. Your body is where you live. In a sense it is *you.* With its many types of cells performing like specialized factories, your body is more like a city full of buildings than like one building. Its cells are full of activity, building and rebuilding, boiling with energy every second. These factories work around the clock, slowing down and

11

speeding up, but not suspending operations even while you sleep.

That I am a scientist should not disturb you; it does not make me a different breed. I am the usual sort of person, no better or worse than my neighbors, with strengths and weaknesses, like everyone I know. Any success that has come my way as a scientist has come because I have learned to emphasize and use my strengths—and because I have been fortunate enough to be at the right place at the right time and to have had some extraordinary experiences and opportunities. Not the least of these is the opportunity to enter into a partnership with you on a project of the widest possible public benefit.

That I can give this help is made possible partly because I have been in a peculiarly fortunate position to learn first hand the basic principles of nutrition. At the same time I have come to grips with vital factors in human nature that have not been fully grasped before. These vital factors are always present.

My principal claim to scientific prominence is that I discovered a universal vitamin—pantothenic acid —without which we and other creatures cannot live. About ten years after the initial discovery, I obtained the vitamin in concentrated form for the first time and made possible and collaborated on its chemical synthesis. I also was involved in concentrating another vitamin for the first time and giving it its name: folic acid. Part of the importance of the discovery and isolation of pantothenic acid is that it helped blaze a pioneer trail: using yeast and other microorganisms, it has been possible to discover other vitamins and learn how they work in living systems. Collecting this kind of information was hastened by decades by using microorganisms, instead of using experimental animals in the traditional way.

Any account of my personal background must

begin with the fact that I was born of missionary parents in Ootacumund, India. My father was a versatile man who preached, taught, designed, and built a seminary with native help, wrote a book in the Telegu language, supervised the casting of the type, bought an old printing press, printed the book, and bound it. (I still have a copy.) In addition, he occasionally extracted teeth for the natives and administered quinine and other medicines.

I presume that I must have inherited, in a very complex way, some of the versatility of my father. Many scientists tend to be highly specialized and very narrow in their interests. Their critics say they come to know more and more about less and less. My tendency is to move away from extreme specialization; this is indicated by the fact that I chose a very broad field—biochemistry—as my principal interest. It covers all aspects of the chemistry of living things. Furthermore, I have made some original scientific contributions in several related fields—medicine, microbiology, botany, pathology, genetics, and psychology.

Nothing in my early training pointed me toward science. School work, except for learning foreign languages from books, was relatively easy and attractive for me. Until the end of grade school, I was a relatively diligent student and sometimes topped my class. In high school and college I was a passable student, but not usually a diligent one. One of my weaknesses is that my eyes do not work together well. I have never been able to read for long periods with pleasure or satisfaction. Since I could not read extensively, I often had to think things out for myself. As a result, I became more of an independent thinker than I would have become if I had used much of my spare time reading. A weakness, thus, turned out to be one of my greatest strengths.

When I went to Redlands, then a small college in California, three subjects interested me: chemistry, literature, and mathematics. After graduating, I went to the University of California at Berkeley. Academically, the year I spent at Berkeley provided me with contacts in chemistry with some of the best minds in the country. It also produced a chance acquaintanceship with an advanced graduate student who was doing research in anatomy. To my provincial, naive mind this was humorous. I had thought that the human body was built thus and so, and that anatomy was a closed book. I suppose I believed, without ever having put my thoughts into words, that every bone, muscle, and organ was pretty much an assembly line product, like the parts of an automobile. While in Berkeley, I began to appreciate that only a small part of the biological world had been explored and that there would always be opportunities for further exploration. It was two years later, that I began exploring, for my doctoral degree, the environments most suitable for the healthy growth and propagation of yeast cells.

One of the most far-reaching insights I gained as a result of this initial study was that yeast cells can be nourished at many levels of excellence. Eventually I learned, from many years of experimentation, that a yeast cell environment can be improved piecemeal—on and on—almost ad infinitum. The better the environment is made, the better the yeast cells perform. I found very early that when individual yeast cells were placed in a limited environment—containing every nutrient then known to be needed by yeast—they grew very little or not at all. (See first photograph, figure 4.) When a very small amount of water-soluble material extracted from plant or animal tissues was added to the yeast environment, a yeast cell propagated as shown in the second picture. The added

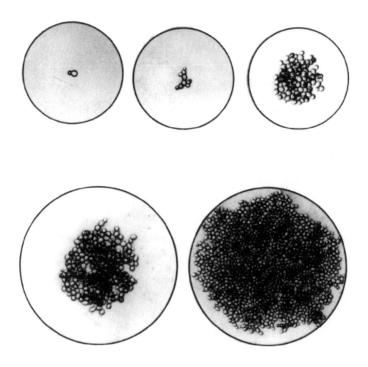

Figure 4. The effects of improving the nutritional environment on yeast cell propagation.

material contained traces of pantothenic acid (unknown at the time) and other nutrients needed by yeast cells for healthy reproduction. When the yeast environment was improved more and more by larger and larger additions of similar extracts, the yeast cells showed their appreciation remarkably, as illustrated in the third, fourth, and fifth pictures in figure 4. Every possible gradation exists between a poor nutritional environment and the best that can be contrived.

Now that you know something about me and my work, we are ready to look further into the wonderful world within you and the kinds of cells that make up your body. As we proceed, I shall be referring to a number of illustrations. All are photographs taken at a magnification of 200—that is 200 times larger than they would appear without magnification. Red cells (erythrocytes or red corpuscles) by the millions are in your blood, pouring through every blood vessel in your body. Disk-like (figure 5), with diameters comparable to yeast cells, they are by far the most numerous of the various kinds of cells you have. At this moment you have approximately 25 to 30 trillion of them. As cells they are unusual in that by the time they reach the bloodstream they have no nuclei and cannot reproduce. After a few weeks they wear out and are replaced by new red cells grown, developed, and matured in the red bone marrow, where up to 10 million new red cells are produced every second. This is one of the many things happening in your body that calls for a continuous supply of nourishing food. Bone marrow, although remarkably productive, cannot produce red cells from nothing. Your blood also contains several types of white blood cells (leukocytes or white corpuscles). Some are pictured in figure 5. They are far less numerous than the red cells.

Liver cells are interesting partly because they reproduce readily. If a portion of your liver were removed surgically, the remaining liver cells would promptly multiply until the organ returned to its original size. If necessary, the body reserves would be called upon for nourishment. This power of reproduction is possessed by many other cells in the skin, bone, bone marrow, and connective tissue. Muscle cells are unusual in that skeletal muscle cells have many nuclei and are in a sense "multi-cells." Compared to other kinds of cells, they are very large; sometimes they are barely visible threads a foot or more in length. Skeletal muscle cells, heart muscle cells, and smooth (involuntary) muscle cells are also shown in figure 5.

Perhaps the most unusual cells in your body are

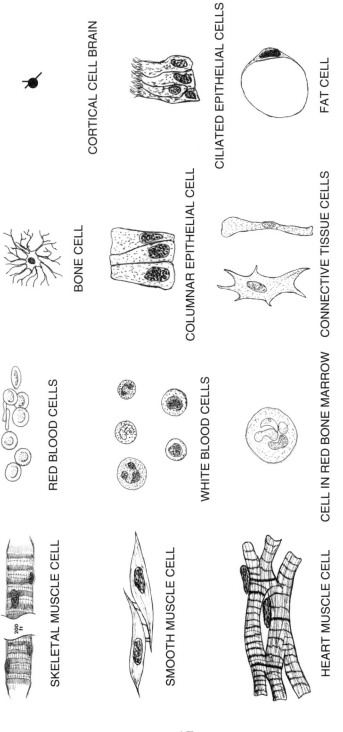

Figure 5. Body cells of various kinds.

CORTICAL CELL BRAIN

CILIATED EPITHELIAL CELLS

FAT CELL

BONE CELL

COLUMNAR EPITHELIAL CELL

CONNECTIVE TISSUE CELLS

RED BLOOD CELLS

WHITE BLOOD CELLS

CELL IN RED BONE MARROW

SKELETAL MUSCLE CELL

SMOOTH MUSCLE CELL

HEART MUSCLE CELL

the nerve cells. Motor nerve cells have a relatively large "head" and a tiny "tail" that may be as long as three feet. Relatively large, tree-shaped cells are among those found in the brain. They are called "Purkinje cells" after their discoverer, and one of them is pictured in figure 6, along with a "pyramid cell," another type occurring in the brain. Other interesting nerve cells terminate in the "rods" and "cones" in the retina of the eye and in the sensory nerve endings in the ear. These endings are pictured in figure 6, along with granule cells from the brain. Numerous tiny glial cells (not shown) are also present

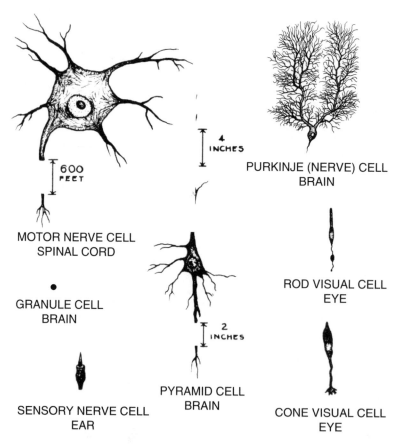

4
INCHES

PURKINJE (NERVE) CELL
BRAIN

600
FEET

MOTOR NERVE CELL
SPINAL CORD

GRANULE CELL
BRAIN

ROD VISUAL CELL
EYE

2
INCHES

SENSORY NERVE CELL
EAR

PYRAMID CELL
BRAIN

CONE VISUAL CELL
EYE

Figure 6. Nerve cells.

in the nervous system.

Reproduction of nerve cells stops at about the time of birth; after that they mature. Their chemistry becomes more complicated; they can repair themselves, but they do not reproduce. When you were a year old, you had as many brain cells as you will ever have. When these die off, as they do, they cannot be replaced. Nerve cells need a great deal of nourishment, perhaps ten times as much as some other cells.

All the cells in your body are involved in everything you do and fail to do. Although the various kinds of cells have many different functions and chemical compositions, all living cells need a good environment and continual nourishment to stay alive, healthy, and active. It may safely be assumed that body cells, like yeast cells, can be furnished environments of many different quality levels: very poor, poor, mediocre, passable, good, and excellent.

The cells in your body often are extremely complicated, not only in composition but also in organization. A liver cell, for example, is more complicated than a watch, a dynamo, a radio, or a television set. It is more like a factory complex. Cells have their own power plants and waste disposal systems. They conduct a multitude of chemical operations and may even build other cells like themselves. They have their own way of designing structures. These include making microscopic "blueprints" and using their own duplicating machinery. They have their own version of the assembly line and also their own intercom systems and devices for receiving messages from outside. Electrical phenomena are incessantly involved in cellular function.

All our activities depend upon body cells and their proper functioning. If we, as human beings, are to perform at high levels of efficiency, our body cells must be encouraged to do the same.

III

GOOD NOURISHMENT:
NATURE'S UNIVERSAL PROBLEM

Can poor nourishment impair a personality? Listen to this. At the Salvation Army in London, England, the behavior and attitudes of seventeen delinquent girls, ages eleven to fifteen, strikingly improved when their diets were improved. The girls had been living on white bread, margarine, cheap jam, quantities of sweet tea, and some canned and processed meats. On this diet, they were quarrelsome and aggressive toward one another and resistant to authority. They also appeared listless and lazy. After their diet was changed to include a variety of fresh vegetables and fruits, dairy products, and fresh meats, the girls underwent a metamorphosis much like Eliza Doolittle's in *My Fair Lady*. Their acne cleared up, their cheeks became rosy, their attitude became more cheerful, and they quarrelled less. Instead of languishing about, bored and listless, they began taking an interest in the world around them and making plans for their own lives.

An experiment with rats, also conducted in England, corroborates these findings under the rigidly controlled conditions possible in animal studies. In this experiment, twenty animals were housed in a large cage and given good nourishments. They got along well together, grew sleek and healthy, and spent considerable time grooming themselves. Twenty other rats were housed in another large cage, but were fed the original diet of the delinquent girls. Within a few days, the animals' hair started to lose its sheen and their appearance began to become dishevelled. The rats became very nervous, biting each other and the cage attendants. As time went on, murder became commonplace. Three animals were killed and eaten by their companions. Eventually, to protect them from one another, these rats were placed in individual cages.

Throughout the entire biological world, obtaining good nourishment is an ever-present problem. Every human being, animal, plant, and bacterium faces it. If this were not so, ridiculous things would happen. Consider, for example, a well-known bacterium, *Escherichia coli*, which grows in your intestinal tract. When this bacterium receives only "good" nutrition, one cell can produce another like itself in an hour; in twenty-four hours, a colony of at least 16 million cells would be produced; in about five days, enough bacterial slime would be produced to bury the earth's surface a mile deep. If such a bacterium were given excellent nutrition continuously, it would accomplish the same feat in less than three days. Of course, such bacteria never encounter ideal nutrition. When they receive meager nourishment they multiply, but soon this nourishment is used up and they have to stop.

In nature's complex and balanced scheme of things, organisms depend on one another for food and also compete with one another for food. As a result, a species or an individual organism often has to "make do" with whatever nutrition is available to it. Often the obtainable nutrition is poor. In the struggle for existence, no organism can at any time automatically be assured of even fair nutrition.

If you live in a part of the country where corn, cotton, soy beans, wheat, or garden produce is grown, you know that crops vary from field to field and year to year. If the temperature is about right and the supply of water and nourishment good, a crop may be ten times as great as if environmental conditions are less favorable. In different parts of the world, crops are growing at 5, 10, 25, or 50 percent efficiency owing to environmental limitations. Similarly, if conditions are right, people prosper; if conditions are poor, they may be miserable. Although you should not answer hastily, it is not too early in our partnership to ask yourself whether human beings sometimes may also be living at similar levels of efficiency and to consider what your own may be at present.

In order to get a clear picture of how our environment affects us and of the role nourishment plays in our lives, let us consider the environment of the moon, on whose surface some of our fellow men already have walked. The moon environment cannot support life: the temperature presents problems and there is no oxygen, water, or food. When Neil Armstrong first set foot on the moon on 20 July 1969, he brought his environment with him.

What are our environmental priorities as human beings? What could an astronaut least afford to leave behind on a trip to the moon? Aside from air pressure to keep his body from exploding in the vacuum and a suitable temperature to keep it from being frozen or cooked, the one thing he needs immediately is *oxygen*. Without this, he would be dead within minutes. We have no store of oxygen in our bodies. The next priority is *water*. This is also absolutely essential; I list it second only because the body carries with it a supply that will last for many hours. However, human beings cannot live even for a few days without an external supply of water. *Body fuel* comes last because people can live—using up their fuel reserves — for many days without an external supply. In the case of the actual moon trip, there was no reason for not supplying it. On the basis of scientific necessity, however, body fuel, though absolutely essential for a long pull, did not have highest priority for a short trip.

In order to make astronauts as comfortable as possible, they were supplied with food providing many other chemical substances such as proteins, minerals, and vitamins, in addition to body fuel. From the standpoint of their immediate physiological needs on the short moon trip, however, the chemical priorities were *oxygen, water,* and *body fuel.*

Now, let's come back to earth. Here we live not a few hours or days or for a few weeks, but all our lives. During our lives, starting from scratch, we have a lot of building, growing, and developing to do, and even after we become adults our body machinery must be repaired, replenished, and kept in working order so we can continue to derive energy from carbohydrates and other energy-yielding food.

We human beings, who live our entire lives on this planet, need to obtain from our environment numerous chemicals that are absolutely essential for the development and continuance of life. Imagine being transported to an environment, otherwise favorable, in which these chemicals are lacking. We would miss oxygen first. If oxygen were to be supplied, the second thing missed would be water. If water also were supplied, the third thing missed would be energy-yielding food. This need could be met on a temporary basis by a sugar or other carbohydrate.

Before discussing other needs, let me clarify what I have just said. Have I indicated that oxygen is most important for life, water is next, and energy-yielding food next? No. *All three* are *absolutely* indispensable to life, but our bodies are so built that their oxygen need must be supplied at least minute by minute, but water and energy, being stored, can be furnished at longer intervals without harm. Animal life cannot continue unless there is a supply of oxygen, water, *and* energy-yielding food.

Included in what we commonly eat are about

forty other chemical essentials. I shall call these *growth and maintenance chemicals*. These, like energy-yielding foods, are stored in our bodies (for varying lengths of time) and do not need to be supplied every minute, every hour, or even every day. *Every one* of these maintenance chemicals also is *absolutely essential* to life and must come ultimately from the food environment. If these chemicals are already stored in the body in adequate amounts, the environmental supply can wait; but if life is to continue, they must be present in our bodies. In infants and growing children they are essential for all growth and development, and in adults they are essential for repairing, replenishing, and keeping in working order the bodily machinery that makes it possible for us to live, derive energy from foods, and do everything we do. These chemicals—along with oxygen, water, and energy-yielding foods—make our lives possible. There can be no substitutes for these essentials.

This group of approximately forty growth and maintenance chemicals is as elemental and basic to nutrition as the letters of the alphabet to language, and more indispensable individually. We can form a great many intelligible words and sentences without using some of the less common letters of the alphabet. Neither our bodies nor any cell in them can function, however, unless *every one* of the growth and maintenance chemicals is present and in place. (The names of these chemicals and the approximate amounts needed daily by an adult are listed for reference in table 1. We shall discuss them more fully later.) All of them are substances we can see, handle, weigh, smell, and taste individually. When observed singly, they are most often in the form of white crystals like sugar or salt; sometimes, however, they are colored, and sometimes they are of an oily consistency. Although each is a tangible, real chemical substance, they often are combined with other substances in foods so that their presence is not obvious. Some are present in foods in tiny (but indispensable) amounts; others are far more abundant. An individual maintenance chemical may make up as much as 1 percent of a food, while others, just as indispensable, may be present in amounts like one-millionth of 1 percent.

The growth and maintenance chemicals are, for convenient classification, often divided into five groups: amino acids, major minerals, trace minerals, vitamins, and other.

The amino acids, when isolated, are white crystalline substances usually obtained from proteins. They are contained in proteins in combined form. Nine of the twenty-odd amino acids present in proteins are growth and maintenance chemicals, and as such are absolutely essential constituents of an adequate diet. They can effectively be supplied separately as amino acids since the proteins themselves and the dozen or more other amino acids found in proteins are not nutritionally essential. These other amino acids can be made within our bodies, whereas the nine amino acids that are among the maintenance chemicals *cannot* be built in our bodies but *must be* supplied in our food.

The minerals needed by the living cells in our bodies are usually present in food in the form of salts. The major minerals are colorless, but some of the ones known as *trace minerals* are colored. These trace elements can be detected in foods only by special methods. When isolated, however, they are perfectly definite chemicals.

The vitamins are a heterogeneous group of substances that belong together only because they are all organic (carbon-containing) maintenance chemicals, not because they resemble one another chemically. There are thirteen vitamins that are well recognized and others that are of doubtful status. In addition, there are two organic maintenance chemicals that do not belong among the vitamins because they are present in foods and in our bodies in relatively large amounts. More extensive discussion of the growth and maintenance chemicals and their presence in various foods will be presented in Chapter XV.

We know that all these growth and maintenance chemicals are essential to continued life as a result of feeding experiments with animals including rats, mice, guinea pigs, hamsters, chickens, turkeys, cats, dogs, foxes, monkeys, cattle, horses, and even fish. Other organisms such as insects, worms, and even yeasts, molds, and bacteria have also yielded important information about the growth and maintenance chemicals needed in human diets. The discovery of pantothenic acid using yeast as a test organism is an example of the way in which this knowledge has been gained. Fortunately, there is a marvelous unity in nature: nutrients essential for one organism are likely to be essential for others.

We know more about the nutrition of rats than that of any other species. The list of growth and maintenance chemicals for rats is the same as for humans, with one notable exception. Rats need ascorbic acid (vitamin C) but, unlike humans, have the machinery in their livers and kidneys to make it.

A series of experiments, simple in principle but not so easy to carry out, will demonstrate the validity of the list of growth and maintenance chemicals for rats. Feed one group of baby rats a suitable mixture containing all the maintenance chemicals listed in table 1. They will develop well. Feed another group of baby rats a mixture containing everything on the list except ascorbic acid. They, too, will develop well. Next, feed all the young rats mixtures from which each of the other maintenance chemicals, *one at a*

TABLE 1
GROWTH AND MAINTENANCE CHEMICALS*

Amino Acids: Histidine (0.7 g), Isoleucine (0.7 g), Leucine (1.0 g), Lysine (0.9 g), Methionine (0.9 g), Phenylalanine (1.0 g), Threonine (0.5 g), Tryptophan (0.25 g), Valine (0.7 g).

Major Minerals: Calcium (1.1 g), Chloride (3.5 g), Potassium (4.0 g), Magnesium (0.33 g), Sodium (2.5 g), Phosphate (3.3 g [1.1 g phosphorus]).

Trace Elements: Cobalt (0.02 mg), Chromium (0.05 mg), Copper (2.2 mg), Fluorine (1.0 mg), Iron (13 mg), Iodine (0.16 mg), Manganese (3.5 mg), Molybdenum (0.15 mg), Selenium (0.06 mg), Zinc (14 mg).

Vitamins: Vitamin A (0.93 mg [4700 I.U.]), Biotin (0.065 mg), Vitamin B_6 (1.8 mg), Vitamin B_{12} (0.002 mg), Vitamin C (60.0 mg), Vitamin D (0.0083 mg [330 I.U.]), Vitamin E (9.3 mg (14 I.U.]), Folic acid (0.19 mg), Vitamin K (0.066 mg), Niacinamide (17 mg), Pantothenic acid (5.5 mg), Riboflavin (1.5 mg), Thiamin (1.3 mg).

Other: Alpha-linolenic acid (1 g), Choline (0.5 g), Dietary fiber (25 g), Linoleic acid (10 g).

* It is suggested that the reader not be concerned, at this point, with details of this list or its nomenclature. These matters will be treated in a later chapter.

See Appendix III for additions and changes in this edition.

---

time, has been omitted. In every case, the rats will fail to develop properly and will eventually die before maturity. How badly they perform will depend on how soon their bodily stores of the missing item are depleted. For example, if iron is omitted, the rats will develop properly for several weeks before the bodily stores of iron are used up, then will show a sharp decline in health. In the case of many of the maintenance chemicals, however, an omission will produce its effects immediately, often in only a few days.

Each species of organism requires a somewhat distinctive set of maintenance chemicals. In experimental animals such as those mentioned above, the lists of maintenance chemicals show strong resemblances to one another. (In some cases, however, the list of maintenance chemicals is not fully known because the nutrition of animals other than rats has not been studied extensively. Indeed, we cannot be sure that we know every item that should be included in the list for rats or the list for human beings.)

Let us turn now to some actual experiments with animals that illustrate how absence or inadequate supply of some of the growth and maintenance chemicals affects life and development.

Vitamin A, as its name suggests, was one of the first vitamins discovered. It was first found essential for the growth and development of rats. The following experiment, however, had to do with high-grade breeding sows. These animals were given a diet deficient in vitamin A early in their pregnancies. In one litter of eleven pigs, every piglet was born without eyeballs. Other abnormalities were also found: cleft palate, cleft lip, accessory ears, arrested ascension of the kidneys. To make sure that lack of vitamin A, and that alone, was responsible for the abnormalities, the researchers later fed the same animals exactly the same diet plus generous amounts of vitamin A. The result was dramatic: in the next litters, there were no abnormalities. (It's interesting to note that rats require about twenty times as much vitamin A for maximum reproduction as they need merely to maintain average health and normal vision.)

Fortunately, it is unlikely that any prospective human mother would consume during pregnancy a diet as free from vitamin A as the sows were given.

The likelihood that a human baby would be born without eyeballs is, for this reason, remote. However, it stands to reason that if severe deficiency of vitamin A can cause such a terrible deformity as lack of eyeballs, a mild deficiency (which often occurs) may well cause less obvious defects, some of which may ultimately produce serious problems.

In another experiment, healthy pregnant rats were fed a mixture of yellow corn meal, wheat protein, calcium, salt, and vitamin D. One third of their young had multiple gross abnormalities. Now, the diet just described compares favorably in quality with the diet of many humans. Whole yellow corn yields energy, protein, minerals, B vitamins, and vitamin A; wheat protein furnishes a respectable amino acid supply. This diet contained some of everything a rat needs, but evidently it did not contain enough of everything. The balance was poor; otherwise, healthy young would have been born.

These two experiments involving pigs and rats help to demonstrate the universal importance of really good nourishment and that this must be furnished even before birth.

These examples will, I hope, whet your appetite for a better understanding of what constitutes good nourishment and why it is not attained automatically merely by eating whatever is offered or appears attractive or merely tastes good. How human beings can obtain good nourishment will be discussed in the next chapter.

IV

HOW CELLULAR METABOLIC MACHINERY WORKS

If supplied with fuel, oxygen, water, and the growth and maintenance chemicals, our bodies can build and maintain complex machinery that runs without interruption for many decades. We should not take this for granted; it is a truly wonderful phenomenon. It is even more wonderful that this building, maintenance, and operation process is repeated with variations in each of the billions of cells that make up our bodies. The total metabolism of our bodies is the sum of all metabolic operations carried on in the cells.

With the help of ingenious biochemists and of microscopes and other special instruments, we have gained spectacular insights into the secrets of cellular metabolism. Each cell operates like a tiny chemical factory. The cells, like life itself, are diverse, vibrant, and full of mystery. As we have seen, there are many kinds of cells; they differ greatly in size and assume shapes like rods, disks, eggs, filaments, pencils, branching trees, long-tailed kites, and other objects. They may even resemble blobs of jelly. To understand what goes on within them, we must learn to think small, to consider the most minute details of cell structure, even the tiny constituent units—molecules—that are far too small to observe even with an ordinary electron microscope.

By far the most numerous molecules in living cells are those of water. Water is a good example of a "chemical substance." Chemical substances are different from mixtures of chemical substances, such as wood, bread, or air. Water can exist in three physical

31

states: gaseous water (water vapor) and solid water (ice), as well as liquid water.

A drop of water may seem to be a small amount, but drops can be broken down into many tiny droplets, each of which is still water (*not* broken down into hydrogen and oxygen). If water is heated, it evaporates into gaseous water, but when condensed by cooling it is still water. In some ways, water is easier to study in the gaseous than in the liquid state. Through refined scientific detective work, we have determined that when one drop of water is vaporized, it is broken into nearly two quintillion little specks of water. (One quintillion is a trillion billion. How large a number this is can better be appreciated if it is realized that a trillion billion *drops* of water would weigh about 50 billion tons.)

Three things about this phenomenon are almost beyond belief: first, that there are so many tiny particles present in a drop of water; second, that scientists can be sure they are present; and, third, that they can count them. Actually, the number of particles (molecules) present in a sample of water or water vapor can be determined with about the same margin of error as that encountered in determining the population of New York City.

I have discussed water molecules to call attention to the fact that oxygen and all the other chemical substances we obtain from our environment also exist as molecules or super-tiny particles. Chemists in the laboratory do not work with single molecules. They deal with amounts that are at least visible. However, when chemists try to visualize how substances are built or constituted, they think in terms of one molecule. (Since all the molecules in a particular pure chemical substance are identical, it follows that if they have visualized one, they have visualized them all.)

Chemists know how the molecules that constitute the chemical substances we obtain from our food are constructed. Many of them are far more complicated in their structure than water. Water molecules each consist of an oxygen atom linked to two hydrogen atoms. Passing an electric current through water breaks it down into these two other substances, each with its own characteristics. Using the customary symbols, the molecular structure is expressed as H-O-H. An oxygen molecule is made up of two oxygen atoms joined together, and its molecular structure is represented by O-O.

In addition to simple molecules of this kind, cells contain hosts of other kinds of molecules. Each cell, however small, has room in it for many billions of molecules—even for billions of protein molecules, the largest kind known. All the growth and maintenance chemicals are present in cells, too, along with many other kinds of molecules that can be produced internally and are not furnished from the environment.

Chemists know precisely what kinds of atoms and how many of each are present in each of the molecules represented by the list of growth and maintenance chemicals (table 1, page 28). Furthermore, they know how the atoms are linked together in each of these kinds of substances. They have this same information about hundreds of thousands of other kinds of molecules, most of which do not occur in our bodies. Protein molecules often contain as many as 4,000 atoms (of at least five different kinds). In a few cases, biochemists have determined just how each atom, of the thousands, is linked in the complex structure. Each protein is different in structure.

All these different kinds of molecules are arranged in an organized manner to make up the "machinery" of metabolism. In these living cells there are no wheels, nuts, bolts, belts, spindles, or gears; yet the machinery built from the various kinds of molecules is so marvelously structured that each type of cell is able to perform its own particular kind of work.

This special kind of metabolic machinery is part of the make-up of all living cells—those in our bodies and other organisms and those in cells that live as separate organisms. When this machinery is operating, energy to make it go is being derived from the burning of appropriate fuels.

The burning of fuel is common to all cells; the process, however, is intricate and not yet fully understood. It takes place smoothly and without friction, at body temperatures. Some warmth is generated, but the operations are accomplished without strong acids, alkalis, or other violent manifestations of energy often used in laboratories.

A key to how this machinery works—and works with such apparent ease—is contained in the word *enzyme*. Enzymes are specially built protein molecules. Merely by their presence, they cause chemical changes to take place rapidly. Each enzyme greatly influences a specific kind of chemical change. Enzymes are built by living cells. The ability of cells to build and use specific enzymes is one of the marvels of cell chemistry.

One enzyme found in cells is carbonic anhydrase. If it is put into soda water it causes the soda water to release carbon dioxide rapidly. The specific chemical change involved here is the decomposition of carbonic acid (H_2CO_3) into carbon dioxide (CO_2) and water (H_2O).

We still do not have a clear or complete picture of how and why such enzymes work. However, the diagram in figure 7 should help you understand an enzyme's role. A protein molecule is a wound-up chain of amino acids linked together. In an enzyme molecule, there are compositional and spatial arrangements that cause it to have on its surface at least one feature that I shall call a "hot" or "active" spot. When a molecule of soda water (carbonic acid) comes near the "hot" spot on a carbonic anhydrase enzyme, the carbonic acid (H_2CO_3) flies apart with incredible speed, forming carbon dioxide (CO_2) and water (H_2O).

Carbonic acid is the characteristic ingredient of soda water which, on standing in the open, eventually becomes flat because of its spontaneous decomposition. It would not be wise to introduce carbonic anhydrase, a white powder, into a bottle of soft drink; the carbon dioxide would be released with explosive violence. In our bodies, little carbonic acid is present in one place at one time; there is no explosion, therefore—just a slow, constant release. The carbon dioxide is carried by the blood to the lungs, where it is released.

In a cell containing millions of carbonic anhydrase molecules, small carbonic acid molecules bounce

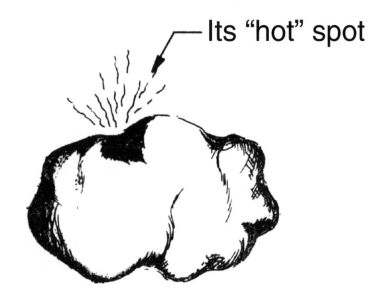

Figure 7. An Enzyme Molecule.

about at great speed—perhaps 1,500 feet per second—and cannot avoid coming close to the hot spots of the carbonic anhydrase molecules. Carbonic acid cannot last long in an environment containing carbonic anhydrase.

Carbonic anhydrase thus carries out a vital function; it causes a release of carbon dioxide which, in gaseous condition, is disposed of when we exhale air from our lungs. A pile-up of carbonic acid or carbon dioxide in the body cannot be tolerated. Breathing in carbon dioxide causes first anesthesia, then death.

Carbonic anhydrase contains zinc as an essential ingredient; without zinc, it has no hot spot and is totally inactive. Carbonic acid decomposes spontaneously (even in the absence of carbonic anhydrase) but far too slowly to take care of body needs. The fact that we need carbonic anhydrase to live is one reason why zinc is one of the maintenance chemicals we need to take into our bodies.

Thousands of other enzymes are known. Another very common one is catalase, the enzyme that causes hydrogen peroxide to break into its basic components—water and oxygen. If, after you have bought hydrogen peroxide at the drugstore, you keep it a long time, it will very slowly decompose into water and oxygen. However, you have probably seen it fizz and bubble vigorously when some of it is placed in the mouth or brought into contact with blood or an open wound or cut. This enzyme is present in saliva, blood, and tissues. When hydrogen peroxide is brought into contact with any of these, a characteristic bubbling takes place. The hot spot on the catalase molecule involves the element iron, without which catalase cannot act. Iron alone will not break down hydrogen peroxide; neither will the protein, without iron. Catalase is produced only when the two are combined in the right way.

Enzymes tremendously speed up chemical reactions within cells; they make possible series of chemical transformations that would be impossible without them. Enzymes do not contribute energy; they act more like extremely effective lubricants. It is important to note that each enzyme has a highly distinctive molecular structure and that each is specific in its "lubricating" action. The enzyme carbonic anhydrase, for example, has no effect on hydrogen peroxide, and catalase does not promote the decomposition of carbonic acid. A particular enzyme promotes only a specific kind of chemical change. The substance affected by a particular enzyme is called its substrate.

Each enzyme is built in a specific way, with active hot spots exposed. When the appropriate molecules come close to these spots, they easily become "disjointed" and chemical changes take place rapidly. The enzyme itself does not change. One enzyme molecule can affect, one after another in rapid succession, millions of molecules of its substrate.

Living cells very commonly burn a fuel called glucose. In this process they use several enzymes. In a way, glucose is "operated on," by first one enzyme and then another. Glucose is modified by one enzyme; the product then becomes the substrate for another enzyme, which brings about another change. Eventually the glucose molecule is fragmented and the separate fragments are transformed through the influence of other enzymes. Although it may seem cumbersome, the process takes place smoothly. The net result is that glucose is burned to produce carbon dioxide and water, with the release of energy that we can use, much as an automobile or motor boat uses gasoline.

When glucose is burned in this complicated way, it yields exactly the same amount of energy as if the same amount were burned in a flame. Millions of kinds of living cells burn glucose. They all go about it in the same general way, using the same kinds of enzymes to bring about the result.

As cells go about their fascinating business, many things are happening besides the burning of fuel. Each kind of cell has its own assortment of enzymes; each cell is a bustling place, building its own structures (including its enzymes), carrying out its own transformations, tearing down and building up its proteins. The most complicated thing a cell may do is reproduce—build another cell resembling itself. During embryonic development, cells even differentiate—that is, build cells different from themselves. This process is still not well understood.

It would be encouraging superficiality if I attempted to discuss the metabolic aspects of reproduction. The reproduction of a mammal involves not only complex genes but also factors that reside outside the cell nucleus. Playing very important roles in the most intricate process are the DNAs (deoxyribonucleic acids) and the RNAs (ribonucleic acids). These are extremely large molecules made up of phosphate groups, sugar groups, and purine and pyrimidine bases, structured in millions of distinctive ways so that millions of DNAs and RNAs are possible, each capable of carrying genetic (inheritance) information.

It's known that brain cells reproduce little or no new cells after birth and yet brain cells fill out and mature during youth and contain, later in life, many minute structures that were not present in the early life of the brain cell.

The numerous activities of living cells call for the use of thousands of specific enzymes built by the cells. Many of these contain not only an assortment of amino acids (giving them a protein structure) but also minerals such as calcium, magnesium, zinc, iron, copper, and molybdenum. Many enzymes and enzyme systems also contain vitamins such as thiamin, riboflavin, pantothenic acid, niacinamide, pyridox-ine, and biotin, all of which are growth and mainte-nance chemicals. No enzyme or enzyme system will work at all if it is incomplete. An enzyme that needs copper or thiamin, for example, will not work even to the slightest degree without the copper or the thia-min.

Let's talk now about *why* all of the growth and maintenance chemicals are essential in nutrition. None of these substances can be built in the body, but many are essential constituents of enzymes that must be built in the body. Many growth and maintenance chemicals, in fact, serve simply as raw materials for the building of enzymes. Elements such as zinc and molybdenum were first found to be constituents of essential body enzymes; this led to a recognition of their indispensability in nutrition.

Adult human nutrition would be vastly different if no maintenance were necessary—if the metabolic machine built in youth continued to run without replenishment. If this were the case, all the mainte-nance chemicals would be superfluous and we would need food only as fuel. Such a situation exists in certain adult insects, such as bees and houseflies. In the earlier stages of development, all the raw materi-als for building metabolic machinery must be fur-nished the insect larvae. During this period, the insects have nutritional needs remarkably like those of mammals. By the time the insects become adults, however, the machinery is built and can function during a short lifetime with little or no maintenance. Adult houseflies and bees thus can live their short lives of a few weeks on practically pure sugar. Mam-mals and many other life forms, however, must al-ways have the growth and maintenance chemicals furnished in their food. Adult humans, unlike adult flies and bees, cannot live by fuel alone. Internal changes are constantly taking place in living cells, and our nutrition must furnish the raw materials necessary for building and rebuilding.

In the total metabolic machinery of living cells are many other substances besides those directly furnished by nutrition; cells produce these, utilizing many different enzymes. Included among these substances are the dozen or more amino acids commonly entering into protein structure but not listed as growth and maintenance chemicals. Also included are the units entering into the make-up of the nucleic acids that play such a large role in reproduction.

Given fuel, oxygen, water, and our growth and maintenance chemicals, a human body can produce with its cells many structural chemicals needed for building metabolic machinery. Chemical formulas for the growth and maintenance chemicals and some of the other substances entering into the make-up of metabolic machinery are presented in Appendix II of this book. The building blocks present in the metabolic machinery of human beings are, in the great majority of cases, exactly the same as the building blocks contained in the metabolic machinery of other organisms of extremely different types: bacteria, yeasts, insects, green plants, fish, reptiles, fowls, and mammals. Of this large number of building blocks, each species is capable of producing its own characteristic assortment—some and not others. The ones that we humans *cannot* produce are those listed as our growth and maintenance chemicals.

The growth and maintenance chemicals are very much alike for diverse mammalian species. Some organisms, however, can produce internally all the amino acids; there are nine we human beings cannot produce. Some organisms can produce many of the vitamins; we can produce none of them. (If we can produce a building block internally, it is not called a vitamin.) No organism can change one element into another. Hence, all organisms need specific minerals and, generally speaking, they need the same ones. For some organisms, the list of growth and maintenance chemicals is relatively simple and consists mostly of minerals; for human beings and other mammals, the list of growth and maintenance chemicals is relatively lengthy. Between these two extremes are organisms whose lists are of intermediate size.

All organisms must build metabolic machinery, taking from the environment *whatever is needed from the outside*. This machinery, which includes a multitude of enzymes, makes possible the utilization of energy by organisms in activities such as building their own structures and reproducing.

V

HOW CAN WE OBTAIN
WHAT WE NEED TO SUSTAIN LIFE
FROM THE ENVIRONMENT?

No one can expect to live long if he disregards the nature of his environment—if he remains naked and unsheltered when a blizzard blows, if he travels unprotected under the desert sun, if he stands his ground when a hurricane approaches. Persons who disregard the quality of their food environment are behaving in the same foolhardy way. The only difference is that the damage done by poor quality food is more sinister and less obvious.

How can we learn to respond to all the demands of the billions of cells within our bodies? How can we make possible the adequate production of all the enzymes that play such a vital role in metabolism? How and where can we obtain from the environment suitable amounts of each and every amino acid, mineral, trace mineral, and vitamin?

The attainment of *perfection* in this regard may be remote, but we all wish to provide ourselves with a good enough internal environment to support us throughout life in reasonable health. Can this be done? The answer is yes. How?

The key to the answer is found in one word: nature. Nature is on our side. This is not a world in which good internal environments are unattainable. In recent decades, many of us have conceived that man's prerogative and destiny is to conquer and subdue nature.

We are following a false god if we forget what Francis Bacon said about four hundred years ago:

"We command Nature only by obeying her." Our fundamental task is to understand nature and learn to live with it and be a part of it. All our problems become clarified when we fathom our own basic nature and that of the world around us. Dr. Albert Schweitzer expressed it philosophically: "The deeper we look into nature, the more we recognize that it is full of life, and the more profoundly we think about it, the more we know that we are united with all life that is in nature."

It is comforting to know that human beings and all earthly organisms share an underlying biochemical unity and that, for this reason, all lives are interwoven. We living things are completely interdependent so far as our nourishment is concerned.

Some of us who live in comfortable city homes and apartments, able to reach into well-stocked shelves of food, may sometimes be tempted to think that we have risen above nature. We tend to forget that the bread that comes from the freezer originates in wheat plants built from soil, water, air, and sunlight. The soil, populated as it is with hosts of microorganisms to maintain its consistency and fertility, is a part of nature. It has a long history of wind and weather, freezing and thawing, and the interplay of many generations of plants, animals, molds, and bacteria. Similarly, we can easily forget that the meat we find packaged in the supermarket came from the soil in the grasslands, where cattle, sheep, and hogs derive the nourishment allowing them to live, grow, and reproduce. When we derive nourishment from meat, we should feel grateful for the living soil, for the plants that nourished the animals, and for the animals themselves, which directly furnish us food.

This relationship is dramatized by the basic fact that the growth and maintenance items we have listed as necessary for human nutrition (see table 1, page 28) are also essential building blocks for the metabolic machinery of every kind of living thing. Because of this, whenever we eat the tissues of plants or animals, we automatically obtain an assortment of growth and maintenance chemicals that will support life.

If, for some outlandish reason, you should follow the idea that zinc is not good for you, or that molybdenum or some other growth and maintenance chemical is to be avoided, this would mean an avoidance of all plant and animal tissues because they all contain these chemicals. One's food would then be restricted to sugar, corn syrup (glucose), starch, and refined fat–items that furnish energy only and lack *all* the growth and maintenance chemicals.

Human beings have the same opportunity to get a life-sustaining diet as do all other creatures. However, we have confused the situation by doing something no other creature has done. We have adopted an arrogant attitude. We have said to ourselves, "We can rise above our biological origin; if we can get our daily bread without physical toil or effort, so much the better." . . . "It doesn't matter about what is in food, just so it looks and tastes good." . . . "If the food we acquire isn't sweet, we can make it so by adding sugar." . . . "If our food doesn't look nice and pink, we can add a little red dye, then it will look rosy and beautiful." . . . "If our food lacks zest, we can remedy this by letting it stand around with yeast, distilling off the juice."

By following this philosophy, we have moved away from the consumption of plant and animal tissues to an alarming degree. Of course, we all eat some plant and animal tissues–otherwise we could not survive–but we continuously eat many "foods" which are, to a large extent, lacking in growth and maintenance chemicals. We are mixed up in our thinking about foods and forget that what we once called "the staff of life" is now very often a staff that has been twisted out of its original shape; that macaroni is not a vegetable; that children do not need energy in the form of sugar; and that poisonous quantities of alcohol cancel the benefits to be derived from wholesome food.

Our animal cousins in the wild state never follow this philosophy, and when we keep them as pets or raise them for food we see to it that they regularly receive high quality food. We have found from experience that food quality makes a tremendous difference in their health. Each of us consumes on the average well over a hundred pounds of sugar a year, yet no one in his right mind would give a pet a corresponding amount of sugar. The food we provide animals is made up of the tissues of plants and animals. For them, we know better than to provide all kinds of processed and refined "foods" that have lost their original character.

When we dilute our own diet with sugar, alcohol, highly milled grains, and processed items that cannot by themselves sustain life, we are short-changing ourselves with respect to the growth and maintenance chemicals.

The quantitative aspects of nutrition are vital. Sometimes I am asked, "How many vitamins do I need?" We need all of them, of course. However, a more vital question is, "How much of each do I need?" It is not difficult to illustrate dramatically how important *amounts* are. If you were to scrutinize the list of growth and maintenance chemicals and decided to consume in one day one *gram* of each of them in addition to oxygen, water, and energy-yielding foods, you would die before sunset because of the poisonous effects, at the level of one gram, of copper, molybdenum, fluoride, cobalt, iodide, selenium, and perhaps some other items on the list. These are needed in milligram amounts or less. If, however, you took it upon yourself to consume daily, in addition to energy sources, only one *milligram* of each of the growth and maintenance chemicals, you would not die right away, but you would lose protein, minerals, and vitamins from your body. Sooner or later, you would become helpless and debilitated. You would be receiving enough of a few of the maintenance chemicals but only insignificant, practically useless, amounts of some others.

When we follow the plan of nature and consume the tissues of plants or animals, we are protected from many of the most flagrant imbalances. This is because there are strong similarities in the metabolic machinery of different species. Certain elements, for example, like copper, iodine, and molybdenum are not only relatively minute constituents of our body cells but also are present in the metabolic machinery of other organisms in very small but indispensable amounts. We call these *trace elements*. Generally, the same elements are found in small amounts in all plant, animal, and bacterial tissues.

The elements present in our bodies in relatively larger amounts, like phosphorus (phosphates), sodium, potassium, calcium, and magnesium, are also present in relatively large amounts in all kinds of plant and animal tissue. Again, if we consume plant and animal tissues, nature protects us from absorbing massive (and fatal) amounts of what should be trace elements and from obtaining only inadequate amounts of the elements we need in larger quantities. No simple rule covers all cases, but there is a tendency for plant and animal tissues to be at least roughly in balance, rather than badly out of balance, as far as the various types of nutrients are concerned.

One of the most important insights into nutrition

has to do with the *amounts* of the different growth and maintenance chemicals we need. There are so many nutrient needs, so many possible levels at which each nutrient may be supplied, so many different kinds of cells to nourish, and so many genetically distinctive individuals involved that in the real world, no matter how or what we eat, *our nutrition is always capable of being improved.* It would be a most remarkable coincidence if one's diet and circulation were perfectly adjusted so as to give every cell and tissue exactly the right amount of each of the forty growth and maintenance chemicals. One's nutrition may be poor, mediocre, good, or excellent, with many intermediate gradations. These gradations in the quality of nutrition probably apply also to the nutrition received by our various organs and tissues—the liver, the kidneys, the heart, and the brain.

If we have an excellent, balanced assortment of growth and maintenance chemicals in our food, the quality of our blood is improved and the cells receive better nourishment. If the heart is better nourished, it works more effectively and blood distribution is improved, thus giving the living cells a better food supply. All of this is perfectly in line with nature's scheme.

In nature, the entire environment is always capable of being improved. Did you ever live in a climate where the temperature day and night, winter and summer, could never be improved upon? What about the humidity, the wind, the rainfall, and the sunshine? Are they ever consistently perfect and not improvable? Did you ever live in a neighborhood where all the neighbors and their dogs and cats were perfectly behaved and always above criticism? Did you ever go to a school where the teachers and students were all perfectly wonderful and without faults?

If we are to live, we must adjust in many ways and

put up with unavoidable imperfections. If the perfect food grew on trees that bore fruit the year round and if there were plenty of trees to go around—one in every back yard and groves for each apartment building—this would be a very different world. In fact, however, we have to exert ourselves to procure food, and since no available food item represents perfection, we can only obtain nourishment that can be rated "good" by diversification and selection. If we are totally ignorant and do not select with discrimination, we can be likened to those who ignore or disregard other aspects of the environment—those who "don't even know enough to come in out of the rain."

The first nutritional experiment I performed illustrates this lack of elementary knowledge. At age twelve, I had the bright idea of buying some baby chicks from a hatchery at five cents apiece and, in just a few weeks, turning them into broilers that I would sell for about forty cents apiece. Alas, it didn't work out. The reason was that I didn't know enough to come in out of the rain, so far as feeding chicks was concerned. Our family had kept chickens for their eggs. I knew that we just fed the hens grain, and that somehow they managed to lay eggs. I didn't appreciate that chick nutrition is far more exacting than hen nutrition. To build new metabolic tissue, chicks need a far richer assortment of growth and maintenance chemicals than hens. Actually, as I now know, baby chicks need a full and generous assortment of about the same growth and maintenance chemicals we human beings need. When I fed those baby chicks grain, they did not thrive and shortly began to die off; it soon became apparent that the whole project was a complete failure. The chicks got an assortment of everything they needed, but it wasn't good enough to foster growth or even sustain life.

My first controlled and more sophisticated nutritional experiment was done about fifteen years later, with revealing results. When I bought some baby rats from an animal dealer in Chicago, he also sold me a bag of grain and seed mixture which, he said, was "just the thing" for rats. I fed them this diet, and they immediately began to gain weight, as babies should. I was not surprised when they gained, on the average, about a gram a day the first week. The second week, I shifted some of the rats to an experimental diet of my own concoction. This, I knew, was deficient in certain respects, but it had one strength—the presence of a good protein source, casein, a prominent ingredient of cheese. Despite the long-range deficiency of this diet, the rats receiving it grew and developed about twice as fast as those on the animal dealer's diet. It became evident to me that the animal dealer had sold me a diet that could be vastly improved. How great the improvement could be was unknown at that time. Now we know that we can feed baby rats so well that they grow and develop in every respect, without becoming at all obese, while gaining five to seven grams each per day.

What about rats in nature? Do they get perfect diets? Adult or partially grown rats are probably lucky if they have access to a good supply of grain of almost any kind—a diet on which they can live and reproduce. But no such supply can be assured. If the entire rat population of the earth consisted of a pair born the same day you were, and if these rats and their progeny had received good food and a good environment continuously, before you finished the second grade at age eight there would be more than enough rats to overrun all the land on earth. There would be one rat for each square foot of land surface.

Although nature doesn't ensure good food for adult rats, it takes far better care of their infants. They get their mothers' milk, which is rich in all the maintenance items except iron. Rats are born with excellent stores of this element, and like human babies, need little of it from the environment during early infancy. In nature, however, mature or partially grown rats "never have it so good" nutritionally as do rats fed in the laboratory by experts.

The principle of the imperfect environment, which applies to all other kinds or organisms, also applies to the species to which you and I belong. Certainly, much of the human race lives with nutrition that is far from optimal. Those who are not starving have to put up with whatever they can get. It is sad to think how many human youngsters, even in "developed" countries, probably receive very poor nutrition and are unaware that good nutrition could make a vast difference in their lives.

We ordinarily do not have to be concerned about certain of our environmental needs. About others, we cannot, if we believe in scientific facts, be complacent.

We get oxygen from the atmosphere and assuming our lungs are working reasonably well we need have no concern for an adequate oxygen supply—unless we start poking our heads into sealed plastic bags or get locked in air-tight refrigerators where the oxygen supply is limited.

Water is another need the supply of which should not ordinarily give us concern. Of course, we may be concerned about impurities it may contain, but an adequate supply is usually available and our thirst mechanism usually tells us adequately when and how much to drink. We do not usually suffer from water deprivation.

In advanced countries, oxygen, water, and body fuel are generally available in adequate amounts. When this is so, nature sees to it that we obtain them. Our breathing mechanisms tell us when we need oxygen, our thirst mechanisms when we need water, and our hunger mechanisms when we need body fuel. If we have a healthy hunger mechanism, it regulates our energy intake.

Your body size (body surface) and the amount of physical activity you engage in determine your calorie needs as an individual. If body fuel is available, you will automatically eat very close to the right amount. If your body size and activity demand 2,500 calories per day, your intake will match this need with considerable precision. If you were consistently to absorb 100 calories extra each day, you would gain weight at the rate of about 12 pounds per year or 120 pounds in ten years. Obviously, nothing like this commonly happens. Of course, some individuals tend to become obese and others tend to be thin, but it takes a very minute consistent error to bring about these results. Millions of people in the United States, for example, automatically, following their own appetite urges, take in—week by week—about the right amount of body fuel in their food. The margin of error over a period of time is usually far less than 1 percent.

Hairsplitting concern for the control of the exact number of calories in one's food is something to avoid. If you have a tendency to become obese, there is probably a very slight defect in your control mechanisms. You may be able to correct this by using "won't power," and possibly you can improve the mechanism itself by careful attention to the *quality* of your nutrition and the proper use of exercise.

Roughage should also not be forgotten. Our diets usually take care of this automatically when we consume a diversified assortment of foods of high quality. However, some individuals may need to pay special attention to this factor.

The matters of real nutritional concern for all of us, however, are the numerous growth and maintenance chemicals, each one of which is essential to life and health. The adequate presence of all these maintenance chemicals in foods is something we cannot afford to take for granted. There are nutritionists who tend to think they can neglect those nutrients with which they are unfamiliar, and that they can take for granted that these will appear in adequate amounts in the foods people generally consume. This is an unscientific view. Unless one has detailed information about exact human needs for all the maintenance chemicals and their quantitative distribution in all foods, one cannot know that neglecting any food is safe. The necessary information on which to base such a conclusion is simply not available. Poor nutrition most often results from the lack of a good assortment of the growth and maintenance chemicals. One can learn good nutrition only by giving attention to *all* the growth and maintenance chemicals.

In the first chapter, we discussed four rats, three of which had been subjected to inferior nutrition. Peewee, the poorest specimen, had access throughout his life to a completely adequate supply of oxygen, water, body fuel, and roughage. What made him so stunted and immature was the lack of a good assortment of growth and maintenance chemicals. Super received such an assortment. This made him a fine specimen.

The desire of each one of my readers, I feel sure, is to obtain superior, in preference to merely passable, nutrition. A more complete discussion of how to attain this goal will be presented in a later chapter. First, we must consider how the fact of your being a distinctive individual impinges on the problem of your nutrition.

VI

MORE ABOUT
YOUR INNER WORKINGS:
INDIVIDUALITY

Although millions of people read their horoscopes each day in the newspapers, astrology usually is not taken seriously by scientifically sophisticated people. Astrology arose in ancient times as an attempt to understand unpredictable individuals and world events. It was well recognized, even long ago, that although newborn babies of the same sex may look much alike, they generally grow up very different.

Astrologers ascribe inborn differences to the influence of the heavenly bodies and the changes in their relative positions. They contend that the progress and outcome of your life is determined by the configuration of the heavens when you were born or conceived. The influence of "stars" at your conception should not be underestimated; however, the real stars in this drama were not the heavenly bodies, but the particular egg cell and the particular sperm cell that joined to bring you into existence.

When you were conceived, the dice of inheritance were cast. Subsequently, chance and other environmental influences entered to modify the development of the person who is now *you*. As babies and small children, we are dependent on parents and other adults for almost all our needs. They make decisions for us and may dominate virtually every detail of our lives. There comes a time, however, when we recognize ourselves as separate entities, taking more and more control over our own destinies. From then on, what happens in our lives depends to a large extent upon us.

A large life insurance company has used the slogan, "Nobody else is exactly like you." This is a gross understatement. Our inner workings make each of us distinctive. If unrecognized, these differences can lead to mistrust and strife; when understood, however, we find each other incomparably more attractive and interesting. Appreciation draws us together. We are far less likely to call each other uncomplimentary names if we appreciate that everyone has a right and even the necessity to be different.

My keen interest in individuality began following a surgical operation I underwent many years ago. Afterwards the doctor gave me a shot of morphine. It knocked out the pain, but I didn't go to sleep as the doctor intended me to do. Instead, my mind became so active that it was racing from one thought to the next. I was then given a larger dose of morphine. All night long, my mind raced faster and faster. I was suffering continuous mental torture.

Why did I react in this way to morphine? The doctor assured me it was merely an "idiosyncracy." Nothing in the library could give me a clue. I had learned, however, first hand and for certain, that in one respect, at least, I was far from being like everyone else.

Since I had to have something in the way of sedation, the doctor tried again, using scopolamine hydrobromide. This gave me sleep—but also, between times, hallucinations. Pictures on the hospital wall became movies. I saw monkeys throwing mud balls at me and squirting blood in my face. I seemed to go on a long automobile ride beside a beautiful seashore. All sorts of crazy things happened to me that the doctor never heard of. Here, again, was an "idiosyncracy," though of a less violent kind. I clearly wasn't just like everyone else in my reaction to these drugs.

The experience aroused my scientific curiosity. There must be a reason for my reaction. However, I was not able to make sense of the puzzle until many years later.

How I came to have some understanding of "idiosyncracies" is a long story. More than twenty years after the morphine episode, a newly published book helped give me insight. This book, *The Atlas of Human Anatomy*, contained, instead of an illustration depicting the stomach, a number of drawings carefully made from autopsy specimens of normal stomachs (see figure 8). On seeing these, I became aware that stomachs differ not only in size and shape but also in the structure and placement of the upper and lower valves. Also, these valves function differently. Furthermore, a Mayo Foundation study published sixteen years after my morphine episode showed that the composition of stomach juices varies much more than stomach sizes. In the case of the pepsin content of the gastric juice, the variation among normal adults is at least a thousandfold. Although pepsin is of some importance as a digestive enzyme, some people manage with very little of it. The hydrochloric acid content of normal gastric juices also varies widely.

We exhibit individuality in *all* our organs. Stomach differences are dramatic and relatively easy to depict. Differences in other organs are often more subtle and intricate, but if we look closely, we will commonly find them. If it were possible to look beneath the surface and see the internal organs and structures in your body and in that of your best friend, we would find that each of you has a distinctive set of internal structures with some marked differences.

One of the most interesting questions you can ask in this connection is this: do normal brains also differ substantially? In 1947, K. S. Lashley, the Harvard neuropsychologist, had this to say:

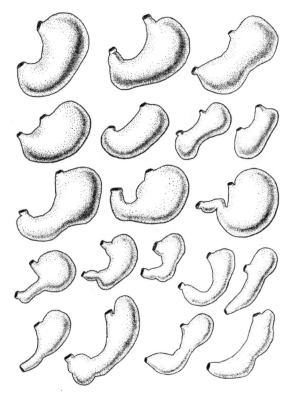

Figure 8. Nineteen stomachs.

The status of the study of variation and inheritance of structure in the central nervous
system may be summarized as follows. The
brain is extremely variable in every character that has been subjected to measurement.
Its diversities of structure within the species
are of the same general character as are the
differences between related species or even
between orders of animals...individuals start
life with brains differing enormously in structure; unlike in number, size and arrange-
ment of neurons as well as in grosser features.

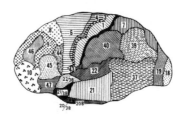

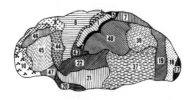

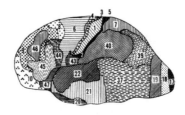

Figure 9. Cytoarchitecture of the three typical human brains (lateral surfaces).

    A. Of the 28 areas represented in these three brain specimens, areas 5, 17, 43 are missing.

    B. Areas 3, 20B, 20/38, 21/38, and 22/38 are missing.

    C. Areas 20B, 20/38, 21/38, and 22/38 are missing.

(from The Structure and Functions of the Brain, S.A. Sarkisov, Indiana University Press, Bloomington, 1966.)

The pictures in figure 9 of the cytoarchitecture (cellular make-up) of the lateral surfaces of three normal brains corroborate Lashley's summary. Although the sizes and shapes of different brain are not very different, the kinds of cells present on the lateral surfaces and their distribution are far from the same. Several types of cells are present in some brains and absent in others. Lashley's study indicates that striking differences occur throughout the brain structure, not only on the lateral surfaces. If I had known this twenty years earlier I might have been able to understand that morphine and other drugs do not necessarily affect all brains in the same way. Here's a question you might like to begin thinking about: do differences in brain structure have anything to do with the fact that people often do not think alike?

Many other parts of the body also have variations in structure. Some have been studied; others are still unexplored. One scientist has studied, intensively, variations in the structure of human lungs.

People exhibit marked differences in the ways they walk, run, talk, breathe, write, read, throw a ball, play tennis, or play golf. Are differences in muscle structure partly responsible? Certainly muscle differences exist. The *Atlas of Human Anatomy* contains an illustration showing different ways in which the minor pectoralis muscle (used when we draw our shoulder down and forward) is attached–sometimes to four, sometimes to three, sometimes to only two ribs. The palmaris longus is one of the muscles in our forearms we use to flex our wrists. Anatomical research indicates that approximately 22 percent of people have peculiarities in the basic structure of the attachment of this muscle. About 13 percent don't have this particular muscle at all. An estimated 1 percent of people have two muscles instead of one.

In figure 10, you can see six arrangements of one specific hand muscle (shown in black)–the one you must shorten to point with your index finger. Notice that when this muscle shortens in hands I and V, it pulls on two tendons and not only causes the index finger to point but also straightens the next finger. Many other muscles in our hands also have distinctive structures.

You and your friends may wish to experiment with your own hand muscles. With one hand partly

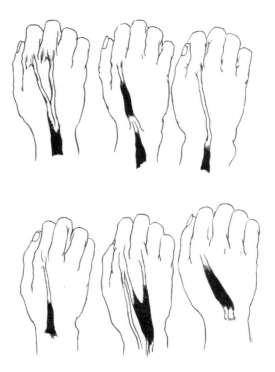

Figure 10. Variations in form and attachment of extensor muscle of the index finger (in black).

closed, see if you can straighten each finger independently of the other. You may be surprised by the differences on this score displayed by members of a small group. If someone in the group can straighten each finger freely without affecting the others, his is an exceptional hand in which the extensor muscle for each finger is attached separately to the appropriate tendon. This test can be turned around; let everyone open his or her hand fully and then try to close each finger without affecting the others.

Hand muscle differences also become apparent when we play the piano or violin, shuffle cards, tie a necktie, write our names, operate a typewriter, hold a golf club, or throw a ball. Hand dexterity is of great importance to a watchmaker and to a surgeon. Although muscle and tendon differences are not the only factors involved in making people's manual skills different, they may exert a very important influence. People can, by persistence, learn to do things that are difficult, but I would strongly advise anyone whose "fingers are all thumbs" not to set out to become a magician or a pickpocket.

It is unfortunate that parents, teachers, and people in general do not routinely recognize the importance of individuality in muscle structure. Robert Schumann, the distinguished composer, suffered sheer misery for years because he did not know about hand muscle differences. This occurred about 125 years before these were recognized and described. Schumann was immensely talented; he composed music when he was only seven years old. He was reared in a family that could provide the best music teachers. He had motivation, and he practiced up to seven hours a day. He could not, however, reach his highest goal: to become the most acclaimed piano virtuoso of his day. The problem was that Schumann had unusual difficulty with some of the fingers of his right hand. We can safely guess that muscle and tendon differences were involved. Schumann tried to invent ways to overcome his difficulties. Some reports even say that he injured his hand in his determination to make it behave. Eventually, he gave up his dream of being a concert pianist. Only then did he turn to composing the beautiful music that made him famous.

Our bodies contain many other distinctive structures and capabilities. Our hearts are distinctive both in structure and in pumping capacity. In "normal" young men, this pumping may vary more than threefold. The branching of our blood vessels is distinctive all over the body. Approximately 65 percent of people have three arteries branching off the aorta, the large vessel delivering blood from the heart. The remaining 35 percent have one, two, four, five, or six branches.

Every individual has a unique system of endocrine glands. These include the pituitary, thyroids, parathyroids, adrenals, the thymus and pineal glands, the sex glands, the pancreas, the duodenal tissue, and the hypothalamus. Each endocrine gland produces and delivers to the blood one or more hormones. (The pituitary yields at least eight.) Hormones are chemicals of widely varying composition, each of which makes possible or greatly influences some vital aspect of body chemistry. They are notably effective in influencing internal energy or drive, appetites, emotions, growth, sex development, sex urge, mental sharpness, and psychological stability.

The endocrine glands, like all other tissues of the body, need continuous nourishment. They cannot manufacture their hormones without raw materials. Usually this is not a special problem because hormone building requires only minute amounts of the various nutrients and these are usually available if the other tissues in the body are being nourished even passably well. In one case, however, hormone building requires a special building block that may be in short supply. In order to build the thyroid hormone, thyroid cells and tissues need iodine. If too little iodine is present, as it is in certain places, then the thyroid gland and the whole body suffer from insufficient thyroid hormone building.

How greatly endocrine systems may vary is indicated by the following facts: In normal people thyroid glands vary sixfold in size; parathyroids, two to twelve in number (approximately 50 percent of people have four), also vary about sixfold in total weight; the testes of males vary about four and one-half-fold in size and weight; the ovaries in females vary about fivefold in size; the "islets" in the pancreas, which produce insulin, vary at least ninefold in number. These variations give a rough indication of the variations in hormone production. The adrenal glands and the pituitary glands do not vary so much in total weight (only about threefold). Since each of these glands produces a number of different hormones, however, the aggregate weights of the total glands are not so significant as would be the variation in the production of the individual hormones. Information concerning the variation in production of all hormones by normal individuals is not available.

Much of the world within you is still unexplored territory. In figure 11 are pictures of seven typical sets of thyroid glands. Notice in one case there are two distinct glands—a pair—and the set pictured at bottom right consists of one large and three small blobs of thyroid tissue. Even if, as sometimes happens, bits of thyroid tissue are found out of place in the body, such bits will produce small amounts of thyroid hormone.

Each individual's endocrine system produces distinctive amounts of the various hormones. You may produce more-than-average amounts of some hormones, less-than-average amounts of others, about average amounts of still others. Each individual has to adapt to his or her own system.

Much that I have learned about human nature since my college days and my morphine experience has come from observing myself and others and conversing with intimate friends. Hundreds of times I have found, in myself and others, evidences pointing unmistakably to individuality in the fundamental make-up of each of us. This is clearly evident in the area of sex. Kinsey's monumental work on sex, with its detailed information and numerous tables, shows that enormous ranges exist among males and females with respect to every aspect of sexual behavior. Sexual

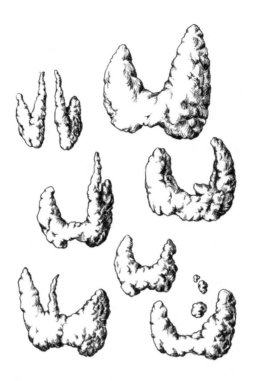

Figure 11. Variation in shapes and sizes of "normal" thyroid glands.

behavior is not simple. It is complex, in that hormones affecting sex are produced not only in the sex glands but also in the adrenals. In addition, powerful hormones that promote sexual development arise in the pituitary. Recognizing that it is impossible to generalize about the "average" or "normal" person's sexual activity helps us to understand how difficult, and important, it is to know yourself as an individual.

This discussion should not lead us to think of our bodies as being made up merely of assorted bits and pieces, each functioning separately. The hormone-producing glands affect one another—this is one of their important functions—and they tend to be interlocked so as to make the body a unified whole.

Another extremely important unifying influence

in our bodies is our nervous system. It is indeed a *system*, in which each part is related to the whole. The nervous system has three basic parts: (1) nerve endings or receptors, which gather the makings of information; (2) the transmission system, which carries impulses; and (3) the interpreting and redirecting center—the brain and spinal cord—which processes these impulses and sends out appropriate new impulses to all the tissues of the body.

The nerve endings or receptors, microscopic in size, are found abundantly in the skin, in the retinas of the eyes, in the hearing mechanisms of the ears, in the tasting and smelling mechanisms in the mouth and nose. A number of these receptors are shown in figure 12. Without these nerve receptors life as we know it could not exist; we would get no messages or impulses whatever from the outside world and would have to remain completely ignorant of its existence.

The body's nerve endings are highly specialized, each kind picking up only certain kinds of sensations. This specialization carries over to the receptors in the skin, which include at least four kinds: (1) those sensitive to pressure, (2) those sensitive to cold, (3) those responsive to the sensation of warmth, and (4) those sensitive to pain. When stimulated, however, they all send out impulses of the same kind. The central nervous system interprets these impulses as a sound, a light sensation, a sweetness, a coldness, a warmth, or a pain, not because of the kind of message received, but rather because of the kind of receptor that sent the impulse.

In ordinary vision, for example, millions of receptors side by side in the retina send impulses simultaneously. The brain interprets these collections of impulses to be a tree, a sunset, or a printed page. We certainly use our eyes in order to see, but we actually see with our brains. An eye detached from the brain

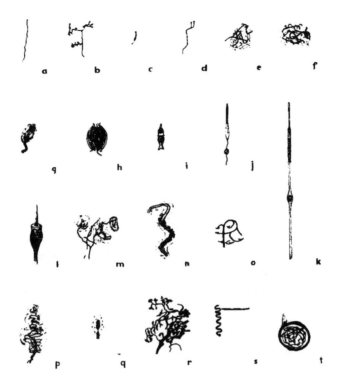

Figure 12. Nerve receptors.

can have images falling upon its retina, but it can perceive nothing. The situation is even more complicated because we have two eyes, and if the eyes did the seeing we would see two trees, two sunsets, or two printed pages. However, since the brain knows how to make sense out of this myriad of impulses, we have what we call binocular vision—that is, vision in depth; farther objects appear farther, closer objects appear closer. If the brain is poisoned by too much alcohol or damaged in some other way, it cannot correctly interpret the impulses from the two eyes and we have double vision. All impulses from the numerous specialized receptors (see figure 12) must be collected and assimilated by the brain before they can have any meaning whatever, either separately or collectively.

Different kinds of microscopic nerve receptors are distributed very widely in different parts of the body. Obviously, light-sensitive receptors are located in the eyes, hearing receptors in the ears, and taste receptors on the tongue and in the mouth. The other receptors are very widely but unevenly distributed. Numerous variations exist in the exact location of individual receptors, so that each individual's sensory mechanisms are "spotted" in a unique way with nerve receptors. The different receptors in the skin are distributed so that there are definite tiny spots, each of which is sensitive to "cold," "warm," or "pain." Study of the skin surface, spot by spot, shows that right next to a spot that is very sensitive to pain is a spot that is completely insensitive to pain but may be very sensitive to warmth or cold. Spots of the same sort are numerous enough, and, hence, close enough together, that if one touches a cold or warm object with one's hand a general sensation of cold or warm ordinarily is felt.

In an experiment to locate pain spots on the backs of twenty-one pairs of hands, the hands were first stamped with ink spots as illustrated in figure 13. Each spot was then pricked mechanically in a uniform way with a standard sharp needle. For each spot the subject indicated one of four responses—"no pain," "mild pain," "moderate pain," or "sharp pain." The results for two of the most contrasting hands in the group are pictured in figure 13. Where the square corresponding to a spot was left blank (white), no pain was experienced. Where the pain was mild, the corresponding square was dotted; where it was moderate, the square was hatched; where it was sharp, it was blackened.

If a score of one is given for each black square, one-half for each hatched square, and one-quarter for each dotted square, the total of the scores obtained from one hand is six and one-half, and from the other (on the right) thirty. The number of "painless" spots on the sample from the first hand is twenty-five and from the second is one.

This experiment proves that nerve receptors are differently distributed in different individuals. Each has a unique pattern. In olden days when witchcraft was believed in, if the hands of a woman who was suspected of witchcraft were found to be insensitive to pain, this brought about her conviction. Relative insensitivity to pain is widespread in the population. Professional boxers have been found who are relatively insensitive to pain, and there have been rare cases of individuals who lacked pain receptors completely. There also are parts of our bodies in which pain receptors are not present at all. Once a surgeon has opened the abdomen, for example, the intestines

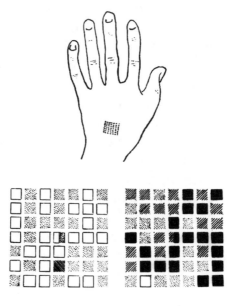

Figure 13. Pain spots on two normal but differing hands. Black spots are highly sensitive; white ones are completely insensitive. The others are intermediate.

can be cut or burned (cauterized) without causing pain. People can have badly damaged internal organs and feel no pain in them. Brain tissue also lacks pain receptors. About 15 percent of people with heart attacks experience no warning pain. The "spottedness" of our nerve receptor distribution causes each of us to have many strengths, weaknesses, and peculiarities in his or her information-gathering system.

In the retinas of the eyes, each of us has a unique distribution of "rods" and "cones." This makes the more sensitive area in the retina (the macula) larger in some eyes than in others. (This probably facilitates speed reading.) Retinal differences permit some individuals, but not others, to discriminate fine shades of color. Because of differences in retinas and the way the impulses are interpreted by the brain, some persons are able to judge with amazing accuracy the speed at which moving objects travel. This ability, possessed in varying degrees, is indispensable for success in baseball, football, tennis, and many other games, as well as in automobile driving.

At least a dozen ways exist in which your visual characteristics may be different from your neighbor's, in addition to the traditionally recognized differences of near-sightedness, far-sightedness, or astigmatism. These involve such phenomena as judgment of motion and speed, depth perception, niceties of color vision, perception in dim light, speed of recovery after exposure to bright light, intricacies of flicker fusion (experienced whenever you watch movies or television), sense of design and proportion, ability to judge and remember how much distance is covered by one inch or one foot, and ability to visualize positions of pieces on a chess board.

Our ears are basically unequal in their ability to discriminate pitches and perform many other feats. When I was a youngster, I heard about and marveled at a child who had a remarkable ear for music; he instinctively knew, in advance, just how every note on a piano should sound. Strangely, I found when I was about eighteen that I possessed this same ability. I could loosen all the strings on a violin and then tune it just as accurately without a piano or pitch pipe as I could with one. I could also play tunes "by ear" on an instrument on which I could learn to play the scale. I know, therefore, that my ears (including the interpretive mechanism in my brain) are different from those of many other people.

Concerning the sense of taste, I have made some original scientific observations. In an article in *Science*, I was credited by psychologists with being the first to point out that the same chemical substance can have different tastes for different individuals. The discovery, made about forty-five years ago, came about when a white crystalline substance was brought to my laboratory for identification. From its origin (it had been extracted from salmon flesh) I suspected that it was creatine, a common constituent of muscle tissue. It had some of the characteristics of creatine, but seemed to differ in one respect. Creatine was reputed to be "a bitter, biting substance." To me and my assistant, it was as tasteless as chalk. Analysis proved, however, that it had to be creatine. We then tested it on our colleagues and found one to whom it had a bitter, biting taste.

About a year later, Arthur L. Fox at the Du Pont Laboratories found that another substance, phenylthiocarbamide, was extremely bitter to some and tasteless to others. Tests on this substance have been extensive. In one study of 6,377 people, 65.4 percent declared it bitter, 21.3 percent tasteless, 5.4 percent sweet, and 4.8 percent salty. The remaining 5 percent called it "astringent," or likened it to lemons, rhubarb, cranberries, or vinegar. How this substance tastes to an individual depends on heredity. Different racial groups show widely different responses. It is most interesting that a person to whom it tastes bitter cannot taste it *unless it is dissolved in his or her own saliva!* On a dry tongue (blotted with filter paper), the substance is tasteless even to one who would ordinarily call it bitter. If dissolved in water, it still remains tasteless to such an individual when placed on a dry tongue. Dissolved in someone else's saliva, it still has no taste.

Fox later discovered that after tasting sodium benzoate (benzoate of soda) some people will say it is sweet, some that it is bitter, others that it is salty, others that it is sour, and still others that it is tasteless. (Those are all the tastes supposed to exist.)

The taste receptors in our mouths are highly distinctive. If any two subjects are tested with a series of substances—it doesn't matter what they are—they will show many different degrees of sensitivity. Many years after the creatine discovery, we found that there were tenfold and even hundredfold variations in the taste responses of different people for different dilutions of such things as sugar, salt, potassium chloride, and hydrochloric acid. Professor Curt Richter of Johns Hopkins University found children who could not taste the sweetness of a 20 percent sugar solution.

The fact that we are all uniquely built is inescapable. We do not see exactly alike, hear alike, or "feel" alike; our tastes are not the same, and the sense of smell is far from uniform in all of us. Idiosyncrasies can now be better understood. Peculiarities in structure and in physiological, biochemical, or psychological functioning are exceedingly common in nature and in the human species. The closer we look, the more we find. Although it may be very difficult to find a complete explanation for a particular aberrant behavior, the widespread existence of idiosyncrasies is in line with the full facts of biology.

Much of the material presented in this chapter has a direct bearing on the problems of nutrition. This is particularly true of the variations in stomachs, intestinal tracts, digestive juices, circulatory systems, the regulatory mechanisms in the brain, the endocrine systems, and the sensory reactions, especially those involved in tasting and smelling. If our bodies were carbon copies of each other, then our nutritional needs would likewise be carbon copies.

The senses of taste and smell appear to be very important factors, especially when we consider that some individuals in practical life depend almost solely on taste and flavor to determine the suitability of food. If a box of chocolates tastes good, this is enough to sell it as a food.

The interplay of the facts of individuality and variability will become more apparent as we get further into varied problems of nutrition in later chapters.

VII

YOUR CRUCIAL HUMAN EQUIPMENT: YOUR MIND AND PERSONALITY

The innate difference we have observed in our muscular, nervous, and endocrine systems, in our intestinal tracts, and in our brains, are structural manifestations of an individuality that transcends these tangible, weighable, and measurable structures–the individuality in our intangible minds and personalities.

Mind and personality are characteristically human attributes. If we lack them, we are not human; if we possess them, we are. Since nutrition affects all of human life, it manifestly affects our minds and personalities. A full grasp of what nutrition can do, therefore, involves a basic appreciation of the nature of our minds and personalities.

Let us now consider how you came to have the mind that is currently working for you. At the time of your birth, your brain had developed almost its full complement of brain cells. Assuming that your prenatal nutrition was reasonably adequate, your brain was now ready to go, but it contained no knowledge whatever. When you first opened your eyes, fuzzy images were thrown on your retina (you had not yet learned to focus your eyes). Your brain received "kicks" from your numerous retinal cells and began trying to make sense out of them. Minute by minute, day by day, and week by week, your brain, receiving endless input from all over your body—your eyes, ears, mouth, nose, and skin—has succeeded very gradually in solving the intricate crossword puzzle presented by the impulses from the outside world. This puzzle-solving process has continued from babyhood until the present and will go on throughout your life. At a rather advanced age, I find that the puzzle is still far from being solved, but I am still working on it, paying particular attention to the parts that already make some sense for me. An interesting aspect of this learning process is that, regardless of the unequal advantages we may have, this development is built on the initial equipment with which we start—equipment that in the aggregate is absolutely unique.

The biological basis of perception compels us to recognize that one's individual "outside world," as registered continuously by the myriad of impulses that reach his brain, is not the same "outside world" that exists in the minds of his neighbors and friends. If a person is blind, for example, the world of color and visual beauty will not be a part of his "outside world." If we have limitations or weaknesses in our eyesight mechanism, we lose part of the visible outside world. The same is true of our other senses. If we have literally "no ear for music," then music is left out of our outside world. If we have weaknesses in our hearing mechanism (which includes the interpretive mechanism in the brain), the world of music is partly blanked out. All of us have plenty of equipment that we can use, however. Even Helen Keller, who was both blind and deaf from early childhood, was able, with the help of her teacher, to build a remarkably attractive outside world for herself. This was possible because of the tremendous capacity of her brain for interpretation. People who consider themselves short-changed so far as equipment is concerned will do well to think of severely handicapped people who have nevertheless lived highly satisfactory lives.

The distinctive detailed structure of your brain is the most important factor in giving you a unique mind. Brains, as we have emphasized, are by no means alike (see figure 9, page 59); all have distinctive patterns; their intricate working cannot be measured in ounces or pounds.

Nature, thus, makes sure that each of us has a distinctive mind. The sets of impulses your brain receives from the outside world are yours alone; furthermore, your interpretive apparatus is unique. Even if the impulses were not unique, your brain would interpret them in its own particular way. When your brain is unable to make sense out of a set of impulses, it tends to neglect them and give its attention to others that it can interpret. If, as a third grader, you had been presented with an algebraic formula, the images of the formula would have fallen upon your retina with accuracy, but the formula wouldn't have made sense and would not have received any attention.

Chemically, your brain is a terrifically busy place. Although your body weighs about fifty times as much as your brain, your brain may use up one-fourth of the total energy of your body. As we shall see more clearly later, your body gets its energy from burning fuel. This burning process takes place all over the body, but about one-fourth of it takes place beneath your skull. The brain has a lot of work to do: gathering impulses, interpreting them, and sending out new and appropriate impulses related to the many operations that take place continuously all over the body. Because of the tremendous job it must do, its nourishment is most important. Brain failure can result from brain malnourishment.

To me, it is astonishing how differently different people perceive the world around them. When I was a youngster I began watching birds build their nests and rear their young. Birds have always been a part of my outside world. Some people, on the other hand, never pay attention to birds—almost never see them or hear them. Their outside world does not, in effect, contain any birds. Some people look at trees and enjoy them; for others trees might as well not exist except perhaps for the shade they give.

I know a man who travelled across the country by train, and said he never bothered to look out the car window at the scenery. Sunsets appeal to some people as magnificent and thrilling; others see them merely as a sign that night will be coming shortly.

Some individuals are not at all interested in how mechanical devices work. When they look at such a device, the appropriate images fall on their retinas, but presumably their brain makes little sense of them, and they turn to other matters. Such people are of course helpless when it comes to making minor repairs or adjustments in such mechanical devices. These devices are not a part of their outside world except as the devices help them with tasks.

Not everyone appreciates gourmet food or fine wines. These are blanked out of their outside world. Poetry has little or no appeal to some people—they never understand it or care to. The beauties of algebra or calculus continually escape some individuals and they are far happier if they never encounter anything of the kind.

Some people can be enthralled looking at snowflakes through a microscope; others would hardly give them a second glance and certainly would not take the trouble to set the stage so that they could be observed. Some children tend to be captivated by watching the phenomena which occur when a piece of wood or coal burns in the fireplace. Others don't care at all just so the heat comes out.

Some years ago, Professor Adelbert Ames, founder of the Dartmouth Eye Institute, demonstrated for me some elaborate experiments that showed clearly that when an image falls on the retina we tend to see that which makes sense to our brain. If an image can equally well be interpreted as nonsense or as something meaningful, we see the meaningful and let the nonsense go. Meaningfulness is based upon previous seeing experience. In accordance with this concept, some individuals are so constituted that such categories of experience as birds, trees, scenery, sunsets, mathematics, machinery, gourmet food, poetry, snowflakes, or even music may have little meaning. Things to which an individual is relatively blind or deaf, thus, receive little or no attention.

It is commonly stated that the brain is the seat of intelligence. This brings up the question: what do we mean by intelligence? Certainly it has to do with all we have learned since babyhood, including what we can do with our minds. There are numerous practical things we can do with our minds. I have made a partial list of forty ways in which a "good mind" can benefit us. We need intelligence to help us (1) remember what happened years ago; (2) remember what happened yesterday; (3) recall dates, names, and telephone numbers; (4) do arithmetic; (5) spell words correctly; (6) use a typewriter; (7) fix mechanical devices; (8) speak English acceptably; (9) write English well; (10) use foreign languages; (11) read books, magazines, and newspapers; (12) play chess or checkers; (13) play bridge; (14) make good grades in school; (15) reason and solve problems; (16) enjoy nature; (17) enjoy literature; (18) enjoy art; (19) enjoy music; (20) enjoy drama; (21) do literary research; (22) do experimental research; (23) understand our own capabilities; (24) understand others and be diplomatic; (25) enjoy and love friends; (26) influence people and get things done; (27) be an effective citizen; (28) find and choose a suitable occupation; (29) select a place to live; (30) find and win a suitable mate; (31) make a livelihood; (32) care for ourselves and our families; (33) choose wisely what we eat and drink; (34) make a good appearance; (35) conserve our money and resources; (36) make inventions; (37) think independently and come up with new concepts; (38) be creative in science; (39) be creative in art; (40) be creative in music.

I made up this list out of my own head; if you had been doing it, your list would undoubtedly be different. Please note, however, that there are forty different things on my list. Although there are overlaps, in general people can be very proficient at doing some things on the list and not at all effective in doing others. Each item, however, involves the use of intelligence, and if one can do any of these things, he is demonstrating a kind of intelligence.

Measuring intelligence adequately is impossible. The I.Q. tests in common use test largely for intellectual qualities that help one make good grades in school. Many of the items listed above, however, are not taught in school, and much of our useful intelligence is not the result of school learning. Ways of testing have not been devised for at least half of the forty items listed. Items involving creativeness, although recognized as extremely important, are not measured in an I.Q. test. Not long ago I was invited to speak at the Annual National Convention of Mensa. This is a group that supposedly prides itself on having members with I.Q.s above some particular level, which I can't remember, and which I think is best forgotten. I delivered the talk and it was well received. Although I was polite enough not to tell them that I thought their mutual admiration society was ill-founded, I did give them some hints about how I feel about measuring intelligence. What I probably had in the back of my mind was this question: How would my listeners' intelligence stack up if their individual intelligences were judged on the basis of such yardsticks as (1) their ability to be diplomatic and make friends; (2) effectiveness as citizens; (3) their performance in selecting suitable occupations; (4) ability to enjoy nature, literature, art, and music; (5) performance in selecting a suitable mate? In any case, my experience over many years leads me to be unimpressed by mere "lesson getters."

In our exploration of the world within you, we have already had a chance to augment our useful intelligence in a number of ways. Look back, particularly, at items 23, 24, 26, 28, 30, and 33. Perhaps you can see how you have already learned things about yourself and others that may help you solve real problems that you have met in the past or that will in the future confront you—problems related to these six items.

If I were hiring a person for a job of almost any kind, I would be much less interested in I.Q. score than in "P.I.C."—his or her *practical intelligence capabilities*. These are abilities of the sort suggested by the list of forty ways a good mind can help us.

Years ago, I invented something called the utopia game which you can use to help answer this question: "Am I, with my supposedly unique make-up, really in a practical sense different from my friends and acquaintances?" If you are, the game will help you know that you are, as well as how you are distinctive.

To play the game, start by reading the following list of twenty-five activities in which you may or may not be interested:

1. *Acting* in plays, etc.
2. Participation in *Athletics*
3. Watching *Athletic* sports
4. Enjoyment of *Beauty*
5. Enjoyment of *Babies* and small children
6. Playing *Card games*

7. Enjoyment of *Carnivals* and similar events
8. *Cooking*, of any kind
9. Having nice *Clothes* (dressing up)
10. Enjoyment of *Eating*
11. Being a *Leader* in activities
12. *Loafing*
13. Contemplation of *Marriage*
14. Enjoying *Medical care* (being nursed, etc.)
15. Having *Membership* in clubs, etc.
16. Enjoyment of *Music*, of any kind
17. *Ownership* of valuable things
18. Enjoyment of *Perfumes* and odors
19. Helping *People* personally
20. *Reading*, of any kind
21. *Religious* worship
22. *Sewing*, of any kind
23. *Shopping*, of any kind
24. *Shows*, of any kind
25. *Travel*, of any kind

Think about each item, how much you like it, and how much pleasure and satisfaction you get out of it. Now, secretly and on your own, put a number after each of the items. If you personally care nothing about an item, mark it 0. If you like it a little and obtain some pleasure from it, mark it 1, 2, or 3, depending upon how attractive it is to you. If there are items on the list that seem very important to you on the basis of the pleasure and satisfaction they give, mark them from 4 to 10, depending on their relative importance. If you have been honest, you will have at least a rough picture of your profile so far as these items are concerned. (If you have made your ratings as though someone were looking over your shoulder, then your ratings are not your own.)

I have played this game many times with students and older people, giving them lists that could not be identified and asking them to make the ratings anonymously. In table 2 are typical results—in this case, those of fifteen high school students. The diversity shown by older people is similar, although the actual choices may differ with different age groups. If you play this game, first make your own secret ratings and, if you wish, compare them with those in table 2. Even if you are in the same age group as the high school students, I will wager that your own personal ratings will show no strong resemblance to those of anyone in that group.

Each of the fifteen students represented in the table is worth taking a look at. Choose any one and try to figure out what peculiarities of muscles or in sensory equipment (eyes, ears, taste buds, and olfactory sense) and mental characteristics, could make him or her give the ratings registered. Can you deduce from your own ratings anything about your own distinctive equipment?

By now, you should be able to take a broad look at yourself. You are not merely the sum of your distinctive nerve receptors, brain, and muscle, circulatory, digestive, and endocrine systems. You are *all* of these and much more, coordinated into a single distinctive individual or person. This all adds up to your *personality*.

Let us imagine for a moment a sandy landscape with no ups and downs, no lights and shadows, trees, rivers, streams, lakes, hills, valleys, or mountains. Not very interesting, is it? Like the landscape, your personality has ups and downs, strengths and weaknesses, distinctive likes and dislikes, unexplored resources.

Nature has made it impossible for you to have a pancake personality, without distinctive form, color, or markings. Nature has made you something like a multicolored distinctive marble—something that can-

---

TABLE 2

STUDENT RATINGS REGISTERED IN
THE "UTOPIA GAME"

		1	2	3	4	5
1.	Acting in shows	0	1	3	1	0
2.	Athletics, participate	2	0	4	0	0
3.	Athletics, watching	3	0	2	2	0
4.	Beauty	2	7	10	1	7
5.	Babies	8	9	3	7	8
6.	Card games	3	2	1	1	1
7.	Carnivals	2	6	6	4	6
8.	Cooking	2	1	1	2	3
9.	Clothes, enjoyment	2	5	2	3	3
10.	Eating	6	4	4	2	2
11.	Being a leader	2	6	2	0	0
12.	Loafing	0	1	2	0	1
13.	Marriage	10	10	8	9	10
14.	Medical care	7	1	7	0	0
15.	Memberships	4	9	0	3	0
16.	Music	2	8	5	1	2
17.	Ownership	2	1	1	0	0
18.	Perfumes and odors	0	2	1	0	1
19.	Helping people	3	8	3	1	2
20.	Reading	1	8	1	0	0
21.	Religious worship	10	10	9	9	9
22.	Sewing	3	0	0	0	0
23.	Shopping	1	1	1	0	1
24.	Shows, all kinds	2	3	3	1	1
25.	Travel	3	3	3	3	1

not be averaged. We can attempt to "average" a group of colorful marbles by mounting them on a disk and spinning them rapidly so that no single marble can be seen. The result: A dirty gray mass with no distinctive color or markings. You are not dirty gray; you are not as flat as a pancake, you have your own personality. This is good.

Philosophers and literary geniuses have known, intuitively or otherwise, of the existence of distinctive human personalities. That personality differences have such a firm, unquestionable biological and physi-

6	7	8	9	10	11	12	13	14	15
0	5	2	0	0	0	0	2	0	0
0	0	0	1	0	1	0	1	0	2
1	1	0	1	1	2	0	0	1	0
1	8	6	1	2	1	1	4	8	5
7	1	7	7	10	10	0	2	9	4
2	1	4	2	2	1	0	1	1	0
3	3	1	4	10	9	8	9	3	0
0	0	8	2	0	0	0	0	2	2
1	3	2	4	3	0	3	2	4	1
1	3	2	6	0	0	2	1	2	2
0	1	2	1	2	2	0	2	3	1
0	3	0	0	0	0	1	9	0	3
10	2	8	8	10	10	10	4	10	8
1	0	0	9	0	0	1	3	7	6
2	0	0	1	2	3	0	1	2	0
3	9	4	2	0	3	2	3	3	1
1	8	1	1	0	0	1	4	6	3
1	2	0	1	2	0	1	1	1	0
8	1	6	5	10	8	3	4	5	6
2	7	3	2	2	2	9	7	6	1
8	0	0	1	3	0	0	3	1	1
0	0	2	10	10	10	10	10	8	8
1	1	3	1	1	0	1	0	1	0
2	6	0	2	2	1	2	2	2	1
2	4	5	2	3	1	1	3	3	2

ological basis is not, however, generally appreciated. Because of this lack of awareness, social scientists have tended to think of people as being much alike, except insofar as they are molded by their environment.

Stuart Chase, a noted writer who had many clear perceptions, became the spokesman for social scientists a generation ago. He (unfortunately) wrote of "George Ratherford Adams" as though he were an average American. He lived in Middleburg, was of average age, height and weight; had a middle income and a medium-sized family. All that was different about him came about because he was molded by his community. Basically, he was thought of as average through and through, and if he had other than a pancake personality it was because of the environment in which he was reared. If people were really like that, everyone raised in a given community would end up having the same tastes. If they played the utopia game, they would all fall into a single pattern. This is a biological impossibility. Of course, people are influenced by their environment, but biologically, even at the start, each has a highly distinctive makeup.

Albert Schweitzer, the famous musician-physician-missionary, himself certainly a man of parts, voiced his appreciation of the complexity of human personality when he wrote: "None of us can truly assert that he knows someone else, even if he has lived with him for years. Of that which constitutes our inner life we can impart even to those who are most intimate with us only fragments; the whole of it we cannot give."

George Santayana, the philosopher, had the same complexity in mind when he expressed the vital truth, "Friendship is almost always the union of a part of one mind with another; people are friends in spots." To me it is perfectly natural and healthy for a person to have several kinds of friends—"baseball friends," "football friends," "bowling friends," "fishing friends," "hiking friends," "bicycling friends," "horse loving friends," "card playing friends," "theater friends," "nature loving friends," "bird watching friends," "rapping friends," "philosophical friends," "scientific friends," "mathematical friends," and whatnot. Friends of many kinds are very seldom rolled into one friend. The hills and valleys of our personalities usually do not agree that well.

The complexities of your personality carry over to

the complexities of your nourishment. There is no capability you have, latent or well developed, that is not affected by the nourishment of the tissues involved. If you are in the process of developing new capabilities, physical or mental, your success will hinge on the quality of your nourishment. What you put into your mouth may make a great difference.

This background of understanding with respect to the uniqueness of our minds and personalities can profitably be borne in mind in connection with the contents of later chapters of this book. Several broad questions will arise. Can your mind and personality be improved by superior nutrition? Might you have potentialities lying undeveloped because your brain cells are not receiving excellent nourishment? Can whole populations be influenced in mind and personality by grossly imperfect diets? Do certain individuals suffer intellectual and emotional damage as a result of poor eating habits while others, relatively speaking, thrive? In deficiency diseases, such as those described in the next chapter, do individuals free from overt disease remain intellectually and emotionally sound?

VIII

LARGE-SCALE
ENVIRONMENTAL ERRORS
FROM HISTORY

With the background of information and insights we have gained so far concerning nutrition and the individuals to be nourished, let us now re-examine and reinterpret some of the nutritional happenings of the past.

Historically, humankind, in its continuous striving for survival, has made several sweeping errors in food selection and handling. As a result, millions of people in different parts of the world suffered for generations from self-inflicted diseases, including scurvy, beriberi, pellagra, rickets, and kwashiorkor. Some of these expensive mistakes were made in an effort to solve the problem of food distribution, which is still acute. Others resulted from an attitude just now beginning to change. Only recently have we been forced to think about environmental problems: we used to take our environment for granted. Today, even in relatively enlightened circles, however, food is seldom seen as an environmental concern. In ages past, this same attitude generated widespread ill health and disease. Then, however, people did not know what we have now learned: that food environments are always of questionable quality and may easily be impaired.

Since prehistoric times, people have had to scrounge for food to stay alive. People in ancient times faced one of the same problems we have today: food is seldom produced exactly when or where it is to be consumed. Hence, means of preservation and of transportation without spoilage had to be devised. Food to be preserved was often dried because foods containing little water, such as dried fish, meat or grain products (hardtack), kept well for long periods. A serious drawback to this method of food preservation–and one that was not recognized before the twentieth century–is that one of the growth and maintenance chemicals is virtually destroyed when drying is done as it was originally, in the presence of air. Nutrition was impaired whenever people ate food dried in this way. Extent of impairment varied from person to person because of differences in physical makeup and nutritional needs. Some who ate dried food for long periods became seriously ill from scurvy and died unless their diet was changed. Undoubtedly, others were damaged to lesser degrees. In the light of modern knowledge, it seems probable that the health and vigor of everyone who ate substantial amounts of dried food was diminished and that to count the number who suffered from scurvy or died is to consider only the tip of the iceberg.

Scurvy, a disease characterized by hemorrhage of the skin and mucous membranes and by spongy gums and debility, was first described in 1260. About 500 years later, a British surgeon, James Lind, seeking to treat British sailors plagued by this illness, showed that the disease had a dietary origin. Dr. Lind advocated the use of citrus fruits, including limes, to prevent scurvy. Today, British seamen are still called "limeys" because they followed his suggestion. It was not until 1932, however, that scientists working with guinea pigs identified the missing link—a definite chemical substance we now call ascorbic acid (vitamin C). This substance is absent from air-dried foods.

Ascorbic acid, as I have mentioned before, is a part of the life machinery of rats, but is not a *dietary* essential for these animals. The same is true of mice, dogs, and chickens. These animals are able to manufacture ascorbic acid from other available chemicals found in food. Among common experimental animals, only guinea pigs and monkeys need dietary ascorbic acid.

By using guinea pigs as experimental animals, scientists have discovered another highly important fact. Although about 0.1 milligrams of ascorbic acid per day will prevent scurvy in a guinea pig, young guinea pigs, for best development, need about fifty times that much. If they receive ample amounts of ascorbic acid—more than enough to protect them against scurvy—several other benefits accrue. They develop rapidly in a healthy fashion; if they are wounded, healing takes place much faster; they are more resistant to lead poisoning; and their immunity system, which helps protect them from infections, functions better.

A very beneficial recent development with respect to vitamin C is the discovery that generous doses of it—far more than enough to prevent scurvy—help greatly to protect many persons from colds. Millions of people have taken advantage of this. Professor Linus Pauling, a Nobel laureate and one of the world's most distinguished scientists, has effectively brought this to public attention in his book, *Vitamin C and the Common Cold.*

Although megavitamin therapy—the use of *large* doses of some of the essential vitamins to treat mental and other disease—is still in its infancy, ascorbic acid is one of the vitamins used in these treatments, and strong evidence indicates that an adequate supply of this chemical to the brain is vital to the prevention and cure of schizophrenia, a common form of mental disease.

The evidence mounts that some persons require far more ascorbic acid than others and that the lack of sufficient ascorbic acid is a common and important way in which people's diets are inadequate. The use of ascorbic acid to promote good development, protect against colds, and help prevent schizophrenia is only a beginning of an unfolding story. Patients with many diseases, including heart disease and the spreading of cancerous growth, can probably be benefited by vitamin C. It would be dishonest for me, as a scientist, to state these possibilities as facts; yet the cumulative evidence that they exist is very strong.

Milling of rice began centuries ago because whole rice stored in hot, humid climates readily becomes weevil-infested and thus inedible. Milled (white) rice is not only more attractive in appearance; it keeps much better. For this very reason, however, it has poorer food value. Because rice is so widely used as a staple food—often an almost exclusive article of diet— its nutritional impairment by milling, as shown in figures 18 and 19, pages 157 and 158, has been one of mankind's most serious large-scale errors in handling the food environment. In regions where white or polished rice was almost the sole article of diet, a disease called beriberi became prevalent. Many nutrients are partially lost when rice is milled, and the nutritional quality of the rice grain is impaired accordingly. One nutrient is lost to such an extent (about 75 percent) that some individuals eating this rice almost exclusively are afflicted with beriberi. This nutrient is thiamin, or vitamin B_1.

If all the thiamin were lost when rice is milled, the nutritional error of milling rice could not have persisted. Without thiamin, people would die promptly, and widespread deaths would have put an end to this practice. Substantial numbers of people, however, can get along on the amount of thiamin they receive when polished rice is virtually their only food. Susceptibility to beriberi varies among individuals in proportion to each person's thiamin needs. These needs vary as much as fourfold. The result was that large numbers who required more thiamin than was available in such a diet died from the disease. In Japan, as late as 1925, beriberi caused 15,000 deaths annually.

Beriberi is a painful and ultimately deadly disease, characterized by inflammation of nerves, paralysis, and general debility. Although only the nervous symptoms accompanying this disease are conspicuous, every cell in the body suffers when there is thiamin deprivation. All metabolic machinery contains thiamin, which is derived from the internal environment. When nervous tissue is incapacitated by thiamin deficiency, all other tissues also suffer.

Another question arises in connection with a diet consisting mainly of polished rice. Do the populations involved suffer also from loss of nutrients other than thiamin? Probably they do, but the effects are more subtle and have not been explored. It seems clear, however, that beriberi mortality statistics constitute a very limited appraisal of the damage caused by extensive use of polished rice.

The interdependence of organisms for their nutrition, discussed in a previous chapter, is exemplified by the contrasting keeping qualities of whole rice and polished rice. Polished rice keeps better and is less likely to be infested by weevils because it has poorer food value and is less able to sustain the life and reproduction of organisms which might infest it.

The milling of wheat as commonly practiced to produce white flour is a nutritional error comparable to that of milling rice, except that white flour has not been used as a sole article of diet and no single identifiable disease has resulted from its use. In terms of deaths produced, the milling of rice has been far more costly than the milling of wheat. In terms of potential impairment of general health and resistance to degenerative diseases, the contrast between the milling of rice and the milling of wheat is probably not so great.

"Enriched" white bread and flour came into existence in the United States about 1940. At that time, some of the nutrients lost in the milling of wheat were restored. The nutrients used since then to "enrich" flour, bread, and cereal products have been thiamin, riboflavin, niacin, and iron. Calcium supplementation was optional. Because of advances in nutritional knowledge, we now know that bread and cereals would be greatly improved in nutritional quality if such available nutrients as pyridoxine, pantothenic acid, magnesium, lysine, and trace elements also were added. General apathy concerning improving the nutritional environment, however, has allowed food manufacturers to remain unaware of or inattentive to recent advances in nutritional knowledge.

Another serious environmental error came about not so much because people wanted food that would be white and keep well, but because in their poverty they tended to depend largely on corn for their food. For human beings, corn has poorer food value than either rice or wheat.

Pellagra developed largely because of the almost exclusive use of corn. Pellagra is characterized by skin lesions (dermatitis), gastrointestinal disturbance, and nervous symptoms. Incidence of pellagra was most prominent in Spain, Italy, Egypt, and the southern United States. In the southern states at one time, an estimated incidence of 170,000 cases, with 20,000 deaths, occurred annually. Of course, this diet impaired the health of many thousands more, but not badly enough so that they reached hospitals or doctors. Nutritional intervention has now almost eliminated overt pellagra in the United States.

Field corn is relatively deficient in two related

growth and maintenance chemicals—tryptophan and niacinamide. If corn were rich in the amino acid tryptophan (which can be converted into niacinamide in the body), pellagra would not develop in those depending very heavily on this food for sustenance. If corn had more niacinamide in it, it would not, of course, be a perfect food, but it would be better, and such dependence on corn would not cause pellagra.

We now recognize that the diets of those who became pellagrous were deficient in several ways and that the nourishment of most of the population in regions where pellagra was prevalent was often very poor. The primary lack in pellagrous diets, however, is niacinamide. This vitamin enters into the construction of a coenzyme present in all cellular metabolic machinery. Thus, in pellagra, as in beriberi, every cell in the body suffers. Because some individuals can get along with less niacinamide than others, not everyone consuming niacinamide-deficient diets contracts pellagra, and because different cells in the body are affected to different degrees by a lack of this nutrient, the symptoms vary from individual to individual.

The symptoms of pellagra are sometimes listed as the four D's: dermatitis, diarrhea, dementia, and death. But these symptoms occur unevenly. Some patients have relatively little skin rash, some comparatively little gastrointestinal disturbance, and some are not mentally deranged. Two closely related facts stand out with respect to pellagra: (1) severe insanity can be caused by a lack of niacinamide; (2) in some cases, this has been cured within forty-eight hours by supplying the missing vitamin.

Is mental disease, generally, caused by some nutritional deficiency or some imbalance of nutrients in the brain? Since there are so many variables in cellular nutrition and so many ways in which deficiencies and imbalances can exist, an affirmative answer to the above question is likely to be correct. It also seems reasonable to suggest that niacinamide deficiency is one of many that can cause insanity. This is supported by the fact that many other specific nutritional deficiencies are associated with mental symptoms, including deficiencies of thiamin, riboflavin, pantothenic acid, vitamin B_6, vitamin B_{12}, biotin, folic acid, vitamin C, iodine, potassium, magnesium, zinc, lysine and other essential amino acids, and glutamine. A further discussion of this is presented in another book of mine, *Nutrition Against Disease.*

The idea that mental disease has its roots in nutritional deficiencies is largely responsible for the development of megavitamin therapy for mental disease. The one vitamin which has been used most often in this therapy is niacinamide (or niacin, its close relative). Because of the difficulties in diagnosing mental disease and measuring its improvement, I have to be skeptical about the clinical results obtained by using this vitamin alone. I am *not* skeptical, however, about the fundamental soundness of Dr. Pauling's orthomolecular approach to mental disease. This involves using substances natural to the brain to treat mental disease. Many impressive successes in the treatment of mental disease with combinations of nutrients have been reported. I have myself observed transformations from severe insanity to complete normality using the nutrient approach, and I have found this very convincing, especially since the rationale behind the treatment seems so sound.

Out of the experience with pellagra has come a new concept of the treatment—and even more important, the prevention—of mental disease. This vital new approach, however, is still in its infancy.

Another historic deficiency disease, rickets, has a complex environmental origin in which food is one factor. It involves, primarily, impaired bone development, and hence is an affliction of the young. If the bones are developing poorly, the whole child's development also is hampered. Rickets does not typically cause the death of children, but some of its victims are deformed as adults.

Rickets is most prevalent in cities in the temperate zone during the winter months when there is least exposure to sunlight. Studying experimental animals that also get the disease has helped to clarify its nature and origin. Rickets can be induced in animals by (1) reducing their calcium intake, (2) reducing their phosphate intake, or (3) limiting their access to sunlight. Scientists made a fundamental advance when they found that experimental animals do not need exposure to sunlight if their food is exposed to sunlight or another source of ultraviolet light. This led to the discovery of the nature of vitamin D, which we have listed as one of the growth and maintenance chemicals.

Vitamin D is unique. In a sense, it does not belong with the growth and maintenance chemicals because it can be dispensed within the diet entirely, provided an adequate (but not excessive) exposure to a source of ultraviolet light is provided. Rickets is clearly an environmental disease; it may be caused, for example, by a faulty physical environment (lack of sunlight) or a faulty nutritional environment (a poor balance between calcium and phosphate or a deficiency of vitamin D in the food). When healthy skin is exposed to sunlight, vitamin D is manufactured from other substances made in the body. Vitamin D is an essential building block in the metabolic machinery of animals, but it may be produced in the skin if ultraviolet light is available.

Long before the nature of rickets was known, cod liver oil became accepted, presumably by trial and error, as a good "medicine" for developing children.

The cod liver oil industry was a substantial one even centuries ago. Cod liver oil is a relatively rich source of vitamins D and A and omega-3 fatty acids, and its folk use was one way in which people managed to improve the environment of growing children without understanding how this was being accomplished.

The problem of rickets has its counterpart today in connection with the healing of bone fractures which, like the healthy development of bones, depends on the proper supply and utilization of calcium, phosphate, and vitamin D (or sunlight). It seems to me that few physicians handle this nutritional problem satisfactorily. I had a friend who, a few years ago, broke his leg. His physician admonished him to stay away from vitamin D. Quite likely as a result of inattention to nutrition, he was unable to walk until months after he should have recovered. For bones to heal rapidly and strongly, the body needs not only appropriate amounts of calcium, phosphate, and vitamin D, but also of every essential maintenance chemical. Bone healing can be greatly speeded up by good nutrition.

Kwashiorkor is a deficiency disease of children. Although it is commonly thought to be caused primarily by a protein (amino acid) deficiency, children suffering from kwashiorkor live on diets poor in many respects. Afflicted children are severely retarded both physically and mentally. Often they are scarred for life by severe malnutrition. Kwashiorkor has been widely observed, but primarily among underprivileged, ignorant, and poverty-stricken people.

The word "kwashiorkor" is derived from an African dialect and means a disease which afflicts a first child as a result of being superseded by a second. Nature provides a baby with mother's milk. However, if a child's nursing period is cut short by the advent of a second baby and there is no effective substitute for the mother's milk, the first child will be severely malnourished. The lesson for us to learn is a striking one. The after-weaning period is the most critical time, nutritionally, in an infant's life. If we wish our young children to avoid kwashiorkor or anything resembling it, we will see that they receive plenty of milk or some effective substitute for it. If children abandon milk and take up soft drinks instead, they are almost certain to be underdeveloped like our rat friends, Peewee and Puny.

These five acute, medically-recognized deficiency diseases—scurvy, beriberi, pellagra, rickets, and kwashiorkor—are mere episodes in human nutritional history. Among more advanced people they are mostly past episodes. Probably even the most short-sighted and unsophisticated among us would agree that we should all guard against these five diseases. A more sophisticated view is that we should *improve the entire nutritional environment since it holds the key to positive health and prevention of disease.*

Advances in nutritional knowledge have virtually eliminated, in the western world, the five scourges I have just discussed. We cannot afford, however, to ignore what is now known about nutrition in the prevention or elimination of such tragic modern scourges as heart disease, mental disease, mental retardation, arthritis, and cancer. So many factors in our nutritional environment can be poorly adjusted and so many human diseases are waiting to be understood that in an enlightened society we must open our eyes to the obvious connection between these two situations. This is not to suggest that disease control is simple—far from it—but the fundamental principle of watching the nutritional environment is simple and far-reaching. Most diseases, "degenerative" and infective, are markedly affected by numerous environmental factors. Like a tree, they have many roots. We need to give expert attention to the taproot—nutritional environment.

IX

NUTRITION BEGINS EARLY

At the moment of human conception, when a microscopic, swiftly swimming sperm cell from the father penetrates a tiny egg cell from the mother, the stage is set for a marvelous nutritional scenario. Parents make possible an infant's human qualities. Distinctive bodily characteristics are transmitted in complex ways from our ancestors. In the fertilized egg cell are the blueprints of a human being; its sex and hundreds of distinctive potentialities are in the planning stage, but the construction is yet to be done. The raw materials must be assembled and integrated gradually over the months in a most intricate way.

Not every building develops according to its blueprints. Intervening events can cause the plans to go awry. The same is true for the blueprints of a human being. If the mother-to-be is very poorly nourished, she may not be able to furnish the raw materials, or she may be able to do so only imperfectly, and the result may be a spontaneous abortion, a stillborn child, a deformed child, a premature birth, or the birth of a mentally retarded infant.

In our bodies, the nutritional environments of cells and tissues, as we have seen, are never perfectly adjusted in every particular and are subject to improvement. This principle also applies to fertilized egg cells and developing embryos. We cannot safely take for granted that the nourishment of a growing fetus will be satisfactory. Nature sees to it that prenatal nutrition is often of high quality, but a fetus cannot develop properly unless the mother-to-be has in her body and furnishes to the fetus, in the fluids that bathe it, a good assortment of food elements—abundant energy-yielding food and *all* of the growth and maintenance chemicals required for the building of metabolic machinery.

Evidence from hundreds of experiments using different kinds of animals shows that nutrition merely good enough to keep adult animals alive will not permit them to reproduce in a healthy manner. Although similar controlled experiments have never been conducted with human beings, the same principle no doubt applies to human beings as to dogs, cats, rats, mice, chickens, turkeys, fish, foxes, and monkeys.

The building of a human baby involves the construction of an intricate brain and coordinated nervous system, a sensory system, a heart and blood vessel network, a digestive tract, a reproductive system, a respiratory apparatus, a blood-forming system, a liver, kidneys, endocrine glands, bones, and muscles. This is an unbelievably complex task—far more complicated, for example, than building a TV set or a skyscraper. Every kind of raw material—every growth and maintenance chemical—is needed in the right amounts at the right time.

Many tragedies occur when nutrition during pregnancy is mediocre or worse. There are nearly 500,000 miscarriages in the United States each year; 125,000 mentally retarded babies are born annually, and many more whose mental abilities are far below what they could have been. It has been estimated that one child in eight in the United States is somewhat mentally retarded. Many other children have malformations, some of which may give no serious trouble at first; years later, the child may wind up in the hospital for surgery to correct some defect. An estimated 50 percent of all children in hospitals are there because of minor deformities.

Many animal experiments have shown that when food is deficient, abnormal reproduction results. In an experiment with rats, for example, scientists found that when given everything else they needed except pantothenic acid (one of the growth and maintenance chemicals) healthy female rats, when bred, produced no young at all. The eggs produced by the female rats were fertilized, and development was started but never completed. When another group of healthy female rats was given a small but inadequate amount of pantothenic acid, 40 percent of the females had young, but half of these were seriously deformed. When still another group was given a larger amount (but still less than optimal), 95 percent bore young, very few of them deformed. From this, we can infer that (1) every growth and maintenance chemical is needed in reproduction, (2) the *amounts* of these nutrients available can be crucial, and (3) individual rats and fetuses vary in their vulnerability to a particular nutritional deficiency.

Experimentation has shown that many different malformations have resulted from a deficiency of folic acid. In some cases, 95 percent of the animals produced have been deformed as a result of *mild* deficiency. (If no folic acid is provided, no young are born.) In rats fourteen kinds of skeletal deformities have been observed to result from folic acid deficiency. The heart and blood vessels may also be malformed. Sometimes animals are born without heads; sometimes the brains are outside the skull; sometimes hormone-producing glands are malformed or absent.

When we realize that these two relatively unfamiliar vitamins—pantothenic acid and folic acid—are essential to reproduction in animals and that deficiencies in these may produce serious deformities, we are led to wonder if deficiencies in human prenatal and postnatal nutrition may not also be responsible for many unexplained defects and deformities. We cannot say with certainty that this is so, but it seems highly probable in light of the fact that we have no scientific assurance whatever that in our society these growth and maintenance chemicals are routinely supplied to human mothers. This hypothesis is also supported by the fact that individual mothers and individual fetuses are vulnerable in different degrees to each nutritional deficiency. A baby may be about average in many respects but, to quote a conservative standard book on nutrition, may "also exhibit some nutritional requirements for a few essential nutrients which are far from average." This highly pertinent fact is one that must be considered in connection with the prenatal nutrition of every infant.

Some women may be able, in spite of inferior nutrition, to produce relatively healthy babies. Some babies, at conception, are more vulnerable than others and cannot withstand mediocre nutrition as well. If only 10 percent of offspring are vulnerable to mediocre nutrition, the problem remains very large. Animal experiments suggest that vulnerability to mediocre nutrition is much higher than 10 percent, and that the diets of many millions are poor enough for their children to be seriously affected.

That prenatal nutrition requires very serious attention is emphasized by two cases that have been brought to my attention recently by Dr. Ruth Harrell, a psychologist. One child was, at nine, a mirror writer and a nonreader. Detailed enzymatic analysis of blood and biopsy specimens devised by Dr. Mary B. Allen, a biochemist of Richmond, Virginia, showed that this boy had some serious nutritional deficiencies, and a regimen of supplementation was instituted. After five days on this program, the mother, herself a physician, called Dr. Harrell to tell of the "miraculous" results.

The mirror writing was gone! After three weeks, the boy, without any special instruction in school, exhibited the reading ability expected of a third grader! It appears that his trouble involved some neurological twist and that the nutrients solved the problem. Although there is evidence that this boy's difficulty had an hereditary base, this did not prevent a suitable nutritional adjustment from being effective.

The second case was that of a boy who still wore diapers at seven, when Dr. Harrell first saw him. He did not seem to recognize his parents or to be aware of his environment. Although he was believed to see and hear, he acted very much as though he did not. He was classed as an idiot. This child's blood and biopsy specimens were also analyzed by Dr. Allen, who suggested a special nutritional regimen to correct specific deficiencies. During the first month, there was only a little improvement. However, when the supplementation was increased—doubled, and in some areas, trebled—the effect was striking and immediate. His mother called excitedly to report that the boy had been "turned on like an electric light." He recognized his parents for the first time, began learning the names of things, and very soon was talking. He now goes to school, reads, and can talk intelligently. Not surprisingly, his intellectual abilities appear spotty, but his I.Q. is low normal.

It is often supposed that an idiot is the result of a poor hereditary beginning and that there is no remedying the situation. The second case suggests that this is not so. While the boy probably had in his inherited make-up some unusual nutritional needs, these could be, and were, met when he was seven years old. If they could have been met during prenatal life, he quite possibly would have been a person of high intelligence. Certainly these two cases of individuals with problems that were very different, yet solvable by nutritional means, suggest very strongly that prenatal nutrition is a tremendously important factor in our lives.

X

INTERNAL NUTRITION

If there is "many a slip between the cup and the lip," there are also many slips further along in the nutritional process. For example, between the actual consumption of good food and the nourishment of all the cells and tissues of the body, there must be digestion, assimilation, and delivery of nutritional elements to the cells. The requirements of our cells are the basis for our need to eat.

Excellent nutrition starts when we put into our mouths good, nourishing foods. However, there are four essential steps to be taken before our body's cells are well fed: (1) *mastication* (chewing), which prepares the food for the second step, (2) *digestion*, which, in turn, prepares for the third step, (3) *absorption*, whereby the digested food is taken into the blood-stream, and (4) *delivery* by blood circulation to brain cells and many other kinds of cells all over our bodies. Thus, there are four different ways in which good food, placed in our mouths, can fail to accomplish its full function. One may waste it by failing to chew it; one may digest it incompletely; one may absorb it poorly; one may circulate it in a faulty manner to the cells that need it. Differences in individual make-up enter into all these processes, none of which is automatically perfect or can be taken fully for granted. A person may have defective teeth or be in too much of a hurry to chew food properly. Our digestive tracts are distinctive, and the digestive process does not always take place with equal facility or thoroughness. Absorption is often a biochemical process involving specific enzymes (not simply a sieve action). Hence, it does not always take place perfectly. Circulation, a most important phase of nutrition, is also greatly influenced by anatomical and physiological differences.

In an average-sized body there are six to eight quarts of blood. As this circulates, it delivers fuel, water, oxygen, and all the maintenance chemicals to the cells and tissues, picks up carbon dioxide and other waste products of metabolism, and delivers these wastes to the kidneys, intestines, lungs, and skin for disposal. As we all know, the heart is the pump; it forces the blood through the blood vessels. A vital part of its work is to pump blood into the heart tissues themselves. The heart, in a sense, feeds itself. Unless its tissues receive an adequate supply of energy and all the essentials of a good internal environment, the heart will fail.

Arteries and veins—the vessels carrying blood to and from the tissues—form a network that resembles a branching tree. Close to the heart, for example, the arteries are relatively large (perhaps as large as one's thumb), but they become smaller and smaller, down to microscopic size, close to the cells they feed. Taking adequate amounts of oxygen and good food to *every cell in the body* is a tremendous undertaking even under the most favorable circumstances. That every cell automatically gets completely adequate service should not be taken for granted. The sizes and branchings of the various parts of the arterial tree are different in different individuals. Blood vessels going to the feet, for example, are much larger in some individuals than in others of the same body size. Because of this, some people are much more prone to have cold feet than others.

While it has not been demonstrated scientifically, it seems reasonable to suppose that, other things being equal, those who have large and ample arteries to the heart are less likely to have heart attacks than those in whom these arteries are relatively small and perhaps malformed. Those who have particularly good circulation to the kidneys probably are less likely to have kidney failure, and those who have especially good circulation to the brain probably have the least tendency to become senile at an early age. These suppositions emphasize the importance of the mechanism for internal nutrition in supplying every type of tissue with oxygen and the needed nutrients. Even if we assume that good food is selected and that it is chewed, digested, and absorbed properly, this is not enough to ensure that adequate nutrients are supplied everywhere they are needed. (If blood circulation in general is ample, however, this tends to ensure adequate distribution.)

As a boy living on a farm, I observed that a litter of pigs would often include a "runt," a piglet smaller and weaker than his brothers and sisters. During embryonic development, the runt was poorly supplied with nourishing blood, and it therefore suffered from generally inadequate nutrition. What happens in a litter of pigs can also happen with similar results within a single developing embryo. If, for example, a blood vessel is formed during development which is too small to feed the growing heart adequately, the result may be a relatively small and inadequate ("runty") heart. Hearts vary in pumping capacity. Poor prenatal nutrition may be responsible for building inadequate blood vessels and, consequently, underdeveloped organs. If hearts can vary in their functional capacities, it is reasonable to assume that other organs—stomachs, intestines, kidneys, livers, and lungs may also vary for the same reasons.

When we speak of differences in the size and branching of the arterial tree in different individuals, we are not speaking of trifling differences. In approximately 65 percent of people, as I have already mentioned, three branches come off the aorta above the heart. In the rest, the number of branches may vary from one to six. Furthermore, the sizes of the blood vessels are such that a blood vessel in one individual may have several times the blood-carrying capacity of the corresponding vessel in another individual.

We are somewhat in the dark as to how all these differences come about, but the fact that in experimental animals nutritional deficiencies during pregnancy can cause all sorts of malformations, including those of the heart, other organs, and blood vessels, suggests strongly that many of the ills suffered by children and adults may be avoided if pregnant women are given the best possible nutrition.

What is past is past, it may be argued. We must, each of us, live with our own individual anatomy as best we can. This is true only to a limited extent. People can, with determination, make their bodies stronger through judicious use of relaxation, exercise, rest, and high quality nutrition. The younger they start, the better their chances of making progress. Probably much of the benefit derived from exercise arises from its effect on the heart and circulation. There are critical times when hearts need as much rest as they can get while pumping away at the rate of almost 100,000 beats per day. In general, however, hearts become stronger if they are taxed but not overtaxed. If we exercise judiciously, the heart is forced to work harder; because of this, it grows stronger and our entire circulation is improved. By exercising, we promote circulation to the lungs, the heart, the kidneys, the digestive tract, and the brain. The importance of good circulation to the brain is difficult to exaggerate. In my experience, nothing promotes healthy mental activity as much as suitable and regular exercise. Because of its delicately balanced and extremely complex functions, the brain is probably more sensitive than any other organ to nutritional deficiencies. Even if the blood is of high quality (which often it is not, because of poor nutrition), the brain cells cannot be adequately fed if the circulation is poor. Anything we can do to improve general circulation will help the brain to obtain what it needs.

We human beings are biological creatures; our whole background for many thousands of years is permeated by the need to move around in search of food, building shelters, and other activities. When and if we become so affluent that we can afford not to exert ourselves—just sit in the shade and eat and drink—our biological inheritance tells us, if we listen, "Get going, and do something, or you will atrophy and die."

One of the advantages of bathing (hot mineral baths, etc.) lies in the fact that this sort of activity promotes better general circulation. When one sprains an ankle or suffers from bruises, one of the most time-honored treatments is to soak the affected part in hot water. This causes increased circulation to the area; this, in turn, brings more ample nutrition and carries away undesirable waste products. Nature does the healing. Should you be so unfortunate as to break a bone in your arm or leg, it is highly desirable that your general circulation be stimulated by whatever exercise you can take. It is also extremely important at this time that you get the best possible food because mending and building bone calls for all the raw materials not only for bone building but for nourishing the living cells that have to do the work incident to the rebuilding. We need to cooperate with nature.

One of the important enemies of good circulation and the resulting poor internal nutrition is a condition called atherosclerosis. This means simply deposits of cholesterol-containing material on the inside of arteries which make them smaller and less able to carry the needed quantity of blood. It used to be thought that atherosclerosis afflicted only those of middle age or older. Now we find that it starts earlier in life. Many young men of military age have the beginnings of this condition.

To prevent atherosclerosis and the poor internal nutrition it promotes, it is necessary to watch one's nutrition. This is a complex problem that is not solved merely by eating less fat or avoiding cholesterol-containing foods. Cholesterol is not a *bad* substance; it is made by virtually every cell in our bodies and is necessary to life. Deposits of it in our arteries are what is bad. If we discard cholesterol-containing foods, we discard the very best foods there are. Although definite scientific knowledge in this area is limited, there is much to be said for the idea that if we eat the right foods and get the right assortment of growth and maintenance chemicals, cholesterol and cholesterol deposits will take care of themselves.

XI

WHAT KINDS OF TROUBLES CAN BE HELPED BY GOOD NUTRITION?

The complexion of the entire world would be changed for many of us if the problems having their roots in poor nutrition could be solved. Frank G. Boudreaux, an eminent New York physician, said in 1960 that nutrition, if really applied, would bring about a greater revolution in medicine than did the discovery that germs cause disease. Many illnesses have their roots in the unhealthy activity of living cells. In biology, we know that if we furnish living cells with a really good environment they exhibit maximum health. This should also be true for the cells in our brains, hearts, intestinal tracts, kidneys, and muscles.

Of course, neither Dr. Boudreaux nor anyone else knows with absolute certainty what can happen before it has actually happened. One can predict only on the basis of accumulated evidence. I am impressed by what Dr. Boudreaux said, however, partly because I knew him to be a conservative, dependable man and partly because his statement was made when we had only about one-fourth as much to support it as we have today.

In preceding chapters, I have presented and discussed many facts and concepts that have a direct bearing on Dr. Boudreaux's remarkable statements. This chapter will present additional supporting evidence.

You have already learned not to expect to attain perfect nutrition in a few easy lessons, even though one may sometimes be surprised by sudden benefits. We can strive for better and better nutrition, and we will be more successful in the future as nutritional science develops.

You have also learned that individual nutrients should not be looked upon as medicines or magic bullets, each curing a specific disease. Nutrients work together as a team, *all* of them entering into the environment of our body cells. Only if one's diet is conspicuously lacking in one nutrient alone does that one nutrient act dramatically because its absence makes impossible the workings of the nutritional team as a whole.

Anemia is a disease that illustrates very well how the nutritional team works. Anemia involves the partial loss of a vital function—the transporting of oxygen to all the cells and tissues. Hemoglobin in the blood is the carrier of oxygen, and in anemia hemoglobin is deficient. It is not surprising that iron deficiency can cause anemia, because iron is a vital part of hemoglobin. Since hemoglobin is a protein and contains all the nutritionally essential amino acids, the lack of any of these amino acids may cause anemia. Anemia can also be produced by lack of copper, vitamin B_{12}, pantothenic acid, folic acid, niacinamide, pyridoxine, or ascorbic acid. These are not present in hemoglobin, but they are essential for hemoglobin building. It is, therefore, a striking fact that one's body cells and tissues may lack *oxygen* because of an inadequate supply of copper, pantothenic acid, or some other nutrient.

Many diseases affect the skin when nutrition is deficient. If one has blotched or unhealthy skin, the internal environment of the skin cells is probably at fault. The skin is more vulnerable to malnutrition than many other tissues because the circulation of blood to the skin cells often is not fully adequate.

In niacinamide deficiency (pellagra), a skin disease (dermatitis) is often present. In biotin deficiency, the skin is also diseased. The first disease recognized as being due to a lack of pantothenic acid was called chick dermatitis. This skin disease, in common with others, is far from being "skin deep." Every cell and tissue in an animal is deficient when the skin cells are.

Many years ago, one of my former students, after he became a physician, experimented with and successfully prescribed vitamin A for the treatment of acne, which can be a very stubborn skin ailment. The fact that vitamin A is not a recognized specific remedy for this condition is owing to differences in the skins of individuals and also to the fact that other nutritional deficiencies may be involved. Certainly acne has nutritional roots.

A professor in one of our leading scientific institutions told me of his own experience with what was diagnosed as psoriasis, an extremely intractable skin disease. On a hunch, he decided to try on himself what were considered at the time rather large doses of vitamin A. After a few months the psoriasis disappeared, but after a trip abroad without his vitamin A capsules, it came back. Not until he resumed taking vitamin A did the condition disappear again. This experience does not prove that vitamin A will, as a rule, cure psoriasis. I would be willing to wager heavily that it will not. What proportion of cases would respond to vitamin A is not known. It may be as low as one in a hundred or even one in a thousand. However, the experience I have related strongly suggests that psoriasis has a nutritional origin.

Eyesight problems may also be lessened or abolished by improved nutrition. A professor of my acquaintance had for years been very sensitive to light and always wore an eyeshade to protect his eyes from overhead lights. Having encountered another individual who had had the same difficulty and had gained relief, I suggested to this man that he try taking five to ten milligrams of riboflavin daily. He followed my suggestion and immediately the trouble vanished. Riboflavin is clearly one of the nutrients involved in maintaining healthy eyesight. This particular individual evidently had riboflavin requirements that were, perhaps, several times as high as those of the hypothetical adult.

A physician once asked my opinion about a remarkable experience she had had with her own eyesight. It had failed so badly she could no longer read with pleasure. This persisted until she began taking several milligrams of extra thiamin (vitamin B1) daily. As long as she did this, she had no further difficulty. All cells in any way connected with vision need thiamin as a part of their metabolic machinery. Apparently this physician had a greater need for thiamin than is considered normal.

Everyone knows that vitamin A is essential for vision. It enters into the composition of the specialized visual pigments that make vision possible. In connection with this, however, a graduate student in science once performed on himself some unusual and unprecedented experiments. Because his color vision was moderately imperfect, he decided to try the effect of relatively high doses of vitamin A on this condition. After careful testing, he became convinced that his color vision improved and deteriorated in direct proportion to his intake of vitamin A, and that for best results he needed far more than the hypothetical adult. A case was recently reported in which many members of the same family had a need for vitamin A perhaps eight to ten times what is considered normal.

The health of the intestinal tract is determined by the kind of environment supplied to its cells and tissues. In pellagra, for example, intestinal tract cells and tissues receive insufficient niacinamide. Diarrhea is a common symptom. Underactivity of the intestinal tract results in stagnation and constipation. Individuals with lifelong constipation problems have found complete relief as long as they furnished themselves extra amounts of pantothenic acid. This vitamin is not a laxative; it merely makes intestinal tissues healthy so that they can do their work. The effectiveness of pantothenic acid in intestinal troubles is corroborated by medical reports of its effectiveness in treating paralytic ileus after surgery. In my opinion, it is unfortunate that many people with elimination problems constantly use laxatives when all they need, probably, is a good nutritional environment for their intestinal cells and tissues.

The use of ascorbic acid (vitamin C) discussed earlier, to prevent and treat common colds is another instance in which a health problem can effectively be handled with better nutrition.

In recent years, dentists have become increasingly interested in the internal environment that comes into contact with the teeth and gums. To build good teeth, all the maintenance chemicals are required; if teeth lack continuous good nutrition, they may deteriorate internally. A remarkable case demonstrating this was brought to my attention by a physician who told me of an experiment in which the needs of a series of individuals for the essential amino acids were being studied. During this experiment (which lasted several weeks), one individual received only a relatively small amount of one of the essential amino acids. Soon she began having serious problems with several of her teeth, and it became obvious that even more serious ones were ahead. The experiment had to be stopped, so far as this individual was concerned. She was given an abundance of the essential amino acid, and her dental problems disappeared. Amino acid, as well as vitamin or mineral, deficiencies can cause serious trouble. Dental problems are often the result of poor nutrition.

Arthritic pain and related disorders probably have a complex nutritional origin tied in with peculiarities of body chemistry. Dr. John Ellis of Mt. Pleasant, Texas, has had remarkable success in treating people with arthritic and partially crippled hands with vitamin B_6. The information reported in a book he has written supports his belief that a great many people are chemically deficient in this vitamin. Substantial amounts of vitamin B_6 are lost when wheat is milled to produce white flour—and are not restored by current enrichment methods. Dr. E. Barton-Wright, in England, has reported his belief that if everyone received twenty-five to fifty milligrams of pantothenic acid each day rheumatoid arthritis would disappear. It is my fear that the situation is considerably more complex than this, but that when medical scientists give the nutritional approach a serious try in arthritis they will have striking successes. The probability that individuals vary widely in their needs for vitamin B_6, pantothenic acid, and other interrelated nutrients is something that must constantly be borne in mind.

One of my former graduate students has advocated the use of pantothenic acid for allergies. Finding that every time he drove across the Arizona or New Mexico desert he had a severe attack of "hay fever," he tried substantial doses of pantothenic acid (twenty milligrams or more) and found that it prevented his allergy attacks. He tested this several times, always with the same results. This observation was turned over to a leading pharmaceutical house, which confirmed that pantothenic acid was beneficial in some cases but that the effects were not uniform enough to warrant a campaign to sell it for this purpose. Since the original observation, this former student has told me that he has found many people who have obtained great relief from allergies from use of pantothenic acid.

A most unusual nutritional result was first called to my attention by an officer of a large New York foundation, and later confirmed by a friend of many years' standing. Two individuals, thousands of miles apart, reported independently that when a nutritional supplement I had devised was used, feet ordinarily prone to be very ill-smelling reportedly became so free of odor that socks worn day after day without washing stayed free of appreciable odor. "Stinking foot disease" is seldom mentioned in medical reports. That it was alleviated by nutritional means in these two cases, however, is a fact. Foot odor is, of course, related to body odor, and it is reasonable, on the basis of these cases, to suppose that this, too, may be affected by nutritional means. The nutritional supplement referred to is a complex one. Whether a different nutrient was primarily effective in each case is, therefore, not known. It can be stated as a fact, however, that malodorous feet can be sweetened by nutritional means.

In earlier chapters, I have touched upon the tremendous potential for improving our mental functioning by means of superior prenatal brain nutrition. We have also discussed the importance of good circulation to the brain and the use of the natural brain chemicals to treat mental disease. Such considerations as these led to the founding in London, in 1971, of the Academy of Orthomolecular Psychiatry. Hundreds of psychiatrists and other physicians are convinced that good brain nutrition is a key to mental health. Many medical reports support this opinion. Niacinamide can cure certain cases of insanity, and I know of one clear-cut case in which folic acid spelled mental health for one who had been seriously afflicted. Good nutrition can also be useful in cases in which some mental functions are impaired. Years ago, a nurse told me that she had taken extra pantothenic acid to stop the graying of her hair, and was convinced that it worked. More important, her memory had been restored most remarkably—a quite unexpected result.

Her memory had begun to fail her after long years of service as an Army nurse. It was so bad that she could easily forget what day of the week it was and would come to work on days when she was not expected, and would absent herself on other days when she was supposed to be on duty. Eventually she was given a medical discharge.

After her discharge, she began taking pantothenic acid for her graying hair and was surprised to find that her memory came back in a most convincing way. After the recovery of her memory, she was a passenger in an automobile accident which later resulted in a lawsuit. Her memory of what happened was perfectly clear, and when she testified in court she was complemented by an attorney for giving a very clearcut story. This nurse had no idea why the vitamin helped her—but she was filled with heartfelt gratitude.

The benefits of pantothenic acid in this case were probably due to an unusually high need for this vitamin in this particular individual. This is not an isolated case, however; pantothenic acid has been found beneficial in the treatment of Korsakoff's syndrome, a condition in which memory loss is involved.

Even our dispositions can be improved by good nutrition. This is not surprising. It is generally recognized that a well-fed baby is likely to be a healthy and good-natured baby, but when the baby's food is unsuitable, he cries and frets. Perhaps we all are like grown-up babies; if we are well nourished we are happier and more agreeable. I have mentioned experiments with animals showing that if they were well nourished they could be housed together, but that poor feeding led to fighting and killing. Although little scientific attention has been directed toward the effects of good nourishment on the dispositions of humans, Professor William Rose of the University of Illinois has told me about some interesting observations in this connection. While doing the classical work resulting in the discovery of the amino acid threonine, he had occasion temporarily to deprive some young men in his laboratory of certain single essential amino acids. As a result, some of them became irritable. Immediately after the missing amino acid was restored, they became their usual amiable selves again. Perhaps some people are irritable because of a high requirement for some amino acid not readily available to them.

When animals are poorly nourished, they become disheveled and unkempt. They cease to groom themselves or to exhibit what we human beings call self-respect. Although it is often noted that patients, once on the mend, begin to pay attention to their appearance, the relationship between grooming and good nutrition has never been studied seriously. It is possible that much of the "don't care" attitude exhibited by some young people today has its roots in poor nutrition.

I became convinced, years ago, that poor nutrition also has a great deal to do with the craving commonly experienced by alcoholics. I found that when experimental animals were well nourished they tended to drink far less alcohol than when poorly nourished. Various specific deficiencies—of vitamin B_1, Vitamin B_6, pantothenic acid, etc.—caused them to drink more, but when the missing nutrient was supplied, their consumption of alcohol often dropped dramatically. These findings led eventually to trials of nutritional supplements in alcoholic humans.

Some years ago, a young alcoholic contacted me for help. Because his was one of the first cases I had dealt with, I could not offer him encouragement. I did, however, give him some nutritional capsules in the hope of filling in some of his serious nutritional lacks. In two weeks he was observed by one of my assistants, whom he did not know, to be greatly improved. The improvement was lasting, and after a year and a half the young man told me that an astounding change had taken place in his life. Before he took the supplement, he couldn't keep from drinking. After taking it, liquor had no particular attraction for him and drinking had ceased to be a problem.

This was not a scientifically controlled experiment. People whose background is such that they see no rationale for the treatment can say that the result came about because of my personality or salesmanship, or that something else led to a change in this young man's life. In the light of my background and experience, however, I think it very probable indeed that the nutritional supplement benefited him by supplying him with adequate amounts of some growth and maintenance chemicals in which he was deficient.

It should be stated that this case is one of many. Although there is a lack of uniformity in response, it should be borne in mind that before this supplement was tried on human beings it had been demonstrated conclusively in numerous controlled experiments that the biological urge to drink alcohol can be controlled by nutritional adjustments.

About the time such experiments were going on, one of my colleagues, Professor William Shive, discovered that glutamine—an amino acid, but not one that is considered nutritionally essential—might be a factor in alcoholism. A physician, with our cooperation, tried this substance on a woman who was a confirmed alcoholic. Since glutamine is tasteless, he was able to put it into her drinking water without her knowledge. After a few weeks she stopped drinking without any other obvious reason; later she got a job and remained sober.

These cases are cited not to support the conclusion that the particular nutritional supplements used will always be effective, but rather to call attention to the strong probability that nutritional treatment can benefit sufferers from alcoholism, especially if it has not progressed too far.

The prevention of alcoholism by nutritional means is in an even stronger position. An adult must usually practice nutritional abuse (in the form of heavy drinking) for several years before he or she becomes an alcoholic. Young (and growing) individuals are more vulnerable. In either case, this nutritional abuse can be prevented if an effort is made *before* the victims lose their will power.

Length of life, and especially length of healthy life, can probably be extended many years through improved nutrition. Linus Pauling, a leading advocate of the nutritional approach to the treatment and prevention of disease, emphasizes that if people were to take ample amounts of extra vitamin C, they would have at any age about one-fourth the usual chance of illness and death. If other supplements in appropriate amounts were used, the benefits would be further increased. A most interesting extension of life span by nutritional means takes place among honey bees. Female worker bees live only a few weeks during the busy summer season, but live longer during dormancy in the winter. When a larva is fed "royal jelly," it becomes a "queen" and may live for as long as seven years and produce during its lifetime tens of thousands of eggs which develop into succeeding generations. What a female bee larva eats during development determines her life span to a remarkable degree. Among other things, royal jelly contains a relative abundance of pantothenic acid. For many years, it was the richest known source of this vitamin. (Codfish ovaries are now the richest natural source known.)

The effect of royal jelly on the longevity of honey bees and its high pantothenic acid content prompted an experiment to test the effect of extra pantothenic acid on the longevity of mice. Two groups of mice were fed the same good diet (a commercial pelleted food) containing what was supposed to be a plentiful supply of pantothenic acid and the other essential nutrients. The only difference in treatment between the two groups was that the drinking water of one group contained extra pantothenic acid. The results showed conclusively that the mice in this group lived about 18 percent longer than the others. In a human being, an equivalent extension would be about thirteen years. Probably some of the mice got enough pantothenic acid in their food, and length of life in these was not affected by the extra amount in their drinking water; other mice, however, were not getting enough and they were sufficiently affected so that the length of life of the whole group was substantially increased. We used mice because their short life span permitted us to complete the experiment in only two years. Presumably, similar results could be produced in many other species, including man, if similar experiments were performed.

I am confident that if human beings were to have their diets supplemented with extra pantothenic acid and other promising nutrients—including, of course, vitamin C—average life spans and health spans would be extended by at least ten years. A substantial part of this extension would be owing to the prevention, by those means, of heart disease, alcoholism, and even cancer.

XII

WHAT IMPROVED NUTRITION
HAS DONE FOR ME

In my youth, when I carried out my baby chick experiment, I was as unaware of the basic facts of nutrition as the majority of people are today. In the course of discovering pantothenic acid, I was very much interested, of course, in yeast nutrition; I also knew, at least vaguely, that this was related to human nutrition. It was in my early forties, however, that I had my first memorable nutrition-related experience, although I did not, at the time, recognize its significance.

I had previously written a book on biochemistry, and the publishers were asking for a revision. I started to work, but immediately became stalled. It was difficult to write anything, and nothing I wrote seemed worthwhile. Quite unlike my normal self, I gave up. A couple of weeks later I began to realize what my difficulty had been; the weather had been rainy and I had failed for several weeks to get adequate exercise. Soon, however, the weather cleared, and I played golf several times. On returning to the writing job, I had no trouble whatever. Evidently my brain wouldn't work properly without exercise. (I now know, of course, that exercise helps to convey good nutrition to the brain.)

In spite of this relatively early experience, it was not until I was nearing retirement age that I began to be seriously concerned with human nutrition. Before that, I had been very much interested in individual vitamins, but I had not looked at nutrition as a whole. On retirement at age seventy, I expected simply to live out the few years left to me as best I could. At that time I developed angina distress due to a heart that couldn't quite do the job of circulating blood to itself and the rest of the body. When my doctor prescribed some pills to take regularly, I told him that I wanted to work on my heart trouble nutritionally, and I began taking vitamin E for the first time.

At about this time, however, I became sufficiently interested in nutrition to write *Nutrition In a Nutshell*, a somewhat unconventional book on the subject. But it was not until about my seventy-fourth year that I began to delve deeply into nutrition and see its enormous possibilities. Up to that time, I had been mildly enthusiastic about nutrition—enough, for example, to take vitamin E for a heart condition— but now I became intensely concerned with it.

The writing of *Nutrition Against Disease* was one of the most illuminating and rewarding experiences of my life. Because of my poor eyesight, it would not have been possible without the help of Rod Thompson, who willingly, even eagerly, spent about two thousand hours in the library searching for related scientific and medical articles. A great deal of thought went into that book, and the most remarkable part of the process was that what I learned about my own nutrition, as I wrote it, made possible its organization and presentation. If I had not gained much insight into nutrition as I proceeded and had not, at the same time, applied it to myself, there could never have been a finished book.

During the writing of *Nutrition Against Disease*, I became fully aware that nutrients work as a team. Hence, I canvassed the entire list of nutrients and tried to make sure that I, personally, was getting everything I needed. Some of the nutrients that gave me special concern were magnesium, vitamin B_6, vitamin C, vitamin E, folic acid, and vitamin A. These and other nutrients were added to my diet in supplementary amounts from time to time. Other individuals should probably be especially concerned about a somewhat different list of nutrients. (I tend not to be introspective. I have kept no record of what I have received nutritionally at different stages of my life. Furthermore, I tend to minimize the importance of what I, personally, consume because I am only one individual and my nutrition should not be accepted as a pattern.)

Since then, as a result of watching my food intake and trying to obtain everything I need, I have undergone a rejuvenation. Before I tell you of this, I must relate an experience which made me appreciate the potentialities of nutritional adjustments more than ever before. While spending the summer in Colorado, I became afflicted with severe leg cramps night after night without exception. I postponed seeing a doctor about this until I returned to my home in Austin, Texas.

When I returned, the doctor whom I hoped to see was on vacation, so I began looking up for myself what I could that might be relevant.

I hit upon the possibility that I might be lacking sufficient calcium. I brought home from the laboratory some precipitated chalk (calcium carbonate) and took a few grams of it. My nightly cramps disappeared the first night and did not return. About this time my doctor returned from his vacation and had my blood analyzed. As expected, the calcium level was relatively high because I had been taking calcium carbonate. I asked the doctor to let me see the analysis because while I had no more cramps, my legs were very restless and uneasy at night. I noted that the phosphate level in my blood was low, although it was still considered "normal." I immediately substituted a calcium phosphate* for the calcium carbonate, and my leg troubles vanished. Clearly I am not the only person who may suffer from this deficiency.

More recently some individuals and physicians have found that vitamin E will abolish nightly leg cramps. For me vitamin E alone didn't work; I had been taking this vitamin when my leg cramps appeared. People's needs are distinctive.

My heart condition was improved. In spite of increased age, I can walk—and carry baggage when I travel—better than I could years ago. My circulation has improved. Ten years or so ago I could not eat a full evening meal without waking up at night with angina distress; now I can. I haven't been awakened at night by angina distress for about ten years. Walking is now my favorite exercise. I can tolerate cool rooms better than before I began seriously studying intensively my own nutrition.

One aspect of my rejuvenation has been something of a disappointment. The circulation (blood vessel supply) in the most sensitive part of my retinas has apparently been marginal all my life, and when atherosclerosis developed (as it always does with age), my eyes began to show the effect. My left eye lost its central vision in about six months when I was seventy-five. This was before I began to give most serious attention to my own individual nutrition. Two or three years later my right eye started to follow suit. It, however, has deteriorated only slowly over several years, and I still can read with my right eye, using suitable magnification. I believe that my improved nutrition has caused a delay in the deterioration of this eye. The most noteworthy sign of rejuvenation, however, has been the retention of the ability and— more importantly, the strong inclination—to do con-

* Cal Pho D (General Nutrition Corp.) is a convenient form in which to take calcium and phosphate.

structive mental work. I believe, in fact, that my mental ability is superior to what it was ten years ago.

In the spring of 1973, before my 80th birthday, I received a letter from a physician-editor in New York suggesting that I write a *Physicians' Handbook of Nutritional Science*. I agreed to do this, and started in June when my wife and I embarked on a trip to Yugoslavia, Italy, and Switzerland. When we returned from this trip, several chapters were already completed, and by Christmas the book was done. This is by far the most effective writing I have ever done on a book. It was by no means a pedestrian job either—it contains much new and provocative material. Writing it was not easy from the standpoint of the amount of thought required. Yet it went ahead like clockwork.

This present book, *The Wonderful World Within You*, has been largely written since the *Physicians' Handbook* was completed. There have been many other activities too, including the writing of a number of serious articles and speeches.

On my 81st birthday it happened that I was in Washington testifying at a Senate Hearing presided over by Senator Edward Kennedy. Some unauthorized person announced my age and the Senator, noting my vigor and posture, remarked to the audience that after the hearing he would find out what kinds of vitamins I was taking.

How long I may be able to continue my activities no one knows, but I still can enter into my work with enthusiasm and vigor. I have no illusions about permanent rejuvenation, but I believe I have discovered an important way to delay the usual effects of old age.

How has all this been achieved? First, I try to concentrate on good foods and have largely avoided poor ones. (The quality of different foods may be judged by the diagrams shown in Chapter XV.) Second, I have taken nutritional supplements. I do not tell other people what they should do, but for me—at my age—I think the use of appropriate supplements is very important. My own choice, as a supplement, is an "insurance" supplement (see page 195), which I have taken since it became available (replacing a somewhat similar one). In addition, I have taken some other nutrients in larger amounts, paying particular attention to the six mentioned on page 128. It is the teamwork of all nutrients that is effective; it is difficult to single out what each one does.

Widely different levels of vitamins A, C, and E are required by different individuals, and since in reasonable amounts they are all harmless, I tend to take generous amounts. The functions of vitamin A (except for vision) are obscure, but it is essential for reproduction and to the health of epithelial tissue. Vitamin C has a number of functions; it protects against unwanted oxidation in the body, helps protect against viruses, and is essential for building collagen, a framework protein (the most abundant protein in the body). Vitamin C must also be very important for proper brain functioning. Vitamin E is also an antioxidant, a fat-soluble one whose prime importance may be in its ability to protect substances vital to metabolism. Vitamin E certainly is useful in preventing undue clotting of the blood, and because of this I have taken it consistently to prevent heart disease. Many different benefits from vitamin E have been reported, all of which may be ascribed to its role in protecting metabolism.

The third thing I do is exercise regularly and judiciously. This, in my experience, is *absolutely essential*. I could not have written *Nutrition Against Disease* or its sequels—*The Physicians' Handbook of Nutritional Science, The Wonderful World Within You*—if I had not walked from two to four miles every day. Such exercise, as I have noted, helps in transporting good nutrition to the brain, where it is conspicuously needed. It has been estimated that, on the average, an adult loses by death and disintegration about two thousand brain cells an hour. Although we start life with many billions of these cells, this loss concerns me. I, therefore, like to conserve brain cells by furnishing them with the best possible environment.

My rejuvenation, finally, is as complete psychologically as physically. I start each day's work with enthusiasm. I have no fears or apprehensions about the present or future. I am blessed with a peace of mind; I rely on a kindly Providence that, according to my experience, moves in mysterious ways to guide and watch over the well-being of those who try to fit themselves into the Divine Plan.

XIII

NUTRITION AND INTELLIGENCE

Intelligence is a many-sided wonder. This was demonstrated by Lewis Carroll who on the one hand was a staid mathematics professor, and on the other the writer of *Alice in Wonderland*, a fanciful story that has been read millions of times all around the world and in many languages.

The mere ability to generate bizarre ideas does not prove that one is intelligent. The ideas have to have an appeal to others before they can be regarded as intelligent.

Many different kinds of intelligence are needed to accomplish anything worthwhile in science, literature, in art, or in music. In each case what is presented must "get under someone's skin" and make its mark in order to be regarded as intelligent. Poetry or art or music which no one likes (or even hates) is pragmatically not poetry, art, or music.

Intelligence is always associated with the possession of a well-developed and extremely complex cerebral cortex in the brain. Animals of different species with similar cerebral cortices are able to take advantage of past experiences to about the same degree. These facts remind me of the progressive appreciation of the complexity of intelligence. L. L Thurstone, an eminent early psychologist, came to the conclusion that there are eight inherited "primary mental abilities" (signs of intelligence) which individuals may possess, each somewhat independent of the others: (1) ability to memorize rote material, (2) arithmetical facility, (3) spatial imagery, (4) word familiarity, (5) manipulative use of words, (6) inductive reasoning,

(7) deductive reasoning, and (8) perceptual and selective facility. Now advanced students of intelligence recognize that this was only a beginning and that our minds really include scores of facets. In other words there are scores of ways in which we as individuals can be "dumb" and an equal number of ways in which we can be intellectually relatively capable. William Lyon Phelps, a famous Yale English professor, used to say, "In mathematics I am slow but not sure."

Man's intelligence is many-faceted and highly complex. Man's cerebral cortex—the seat of his intelligence—is also extremely complex. If we are to relate nutrition to intelligence, we must therefore be concerned with the nutrition of the cerebral cortex.

A striking finding has been made in recent years —namely, that in rats the size and development of the cerebral cortex can be greatly modified by prenatal nutrition. If pregnant rats are consistently deprived of an adequate amount of food, the brains of the young are adversely affected and cell counts in their brains are lower than when their mothers have received a good supply of food.

Other experiments with rats also reinforce the importance of nutrition to the brain. Taking advantage of peculiarities in rat anatomy, it is possible by relatively minor surgery to produce a female rat which will produce a "half litter" of young. When these prospective mothers are fed well, the developing baby rats have access to a much better blood supply and, therefore, to more ample nutrition than if a normal litter were being supported. As a result, the individual rats in such litters at birth have weighed a little more than those from full litters. More striking, however, have been the 10 to 15 percent increase in the weight of the cerebral cortex and similar increases in brain cell counts.

In rats, cell multiplication in the brain continues

for about three weeks after birth. Presumably rats from a large litter could, if given excellent, abundant nutrition during this period, at least partly make up for what they didn't get during their life in the uterus. However, if rats from a small litter were also given excellent, abundant nutrition during the same period, they should probably still be ahead of the large-litter rats at weaning. The advantage would probably continue throughout life. These findings emphasize that brains are built in a superior way if plentiful and abundantly adequate nourishment is supplied. This, of course, applies to humans as well as to rats.

In humans, brain cell multiplication also continues for a time after birth. After the cells stop multiplying, development, maturation, and growth in bulk of the brain cells continue as long as the individual grows. A baby whose brain development was hampered by inadequate or unbalanced nutrition during the gestation period can doubtless be helped tremendously by excellent and fully adequate nutrition during the entire growing period of about twenty years. Of course, if brain development is superior at the start, so much the better. And because early stages of brain development are crucial, nothing can be done to overcome the setback completely if early development is much retarded.

Other relatively recent studies have shown that the full development of the cerebral cortex of an animal requires not only good and ample prenatal and postnatal nutrition but also learning opportunities. It was found that when two groups of rats were treated differently in this respect—one group was kept in isolated cages where they could only eat and sleep; the other group was given many playthings in their cages—the rats with better learning opportunities developed larger cerebral cortices.

These experiments constitute concrete support

for the idea that if children are given an opportunity to use their heads the result will be a substantial increase in the size of the cerebral cortex and an increase in intelligence. If educational opportunities are given, but the individual child is not adequately furnished with the raw material necessary for building up the cerebral cortex, underdevelopment still results, just as it does when no learning opportunities are provided. A child needs continuously two things: food for thought and food for building the cerebral cortex.

Chemically, the brain is an extremely active part of the body. Even at rest, our bodies use (on the average) perhaps 320 liters of pure oxygen gas each day. Liquefied, this would be about two cupfuls and would weigh approximately one pound. Of this, one-fifth is needed by the brain. By weight, this is about ten times its share. The brain gets this amount of oxygen because it needs it and uses it up. The amount of chemical burning that takes place in the brain is tremendous and requires the functioning of metabolic machinery, which must be built and maintained. This is why the nutrition of the brain is so important and why nutrition is so indispensable for the development of intelligence.

XIV

POLLUTION OF
OUR INTERNAL ENVIRONMENTS

Some pollution of our air and water, and consequently our internal environments, is inevitable and has been with us ever since human beings began to populate this planet. This is one of the imperfections in our environment to which we have become accustomed. When population becomes more dense, however, pollution increases and, especially if we are careless, can become dangerous and damaging. Even pollution of food, which results in pollution of our internal environments, is not a new problem. However, it takes on new forms and becomes more serious in industrial societies where foods are extensively processed into convenient forms that can be packaged, kept for long periods, and shipped long distances.

Pollution of any kind must always be evaluated both qualitatively and quantitatively: we must consider first, *what* pollutants exist and second, *how much* of the pollutants are involved.

Qualitatively, even the purest air contains traces of such substances as carbon monoxide, sulfur dioxide, and oxides of nitrogen, ozone, hydrogen sulfide, and methane. These undesirable substances were present in the air even in prehistoric times; they had their origin in volcanoes, sulfur springs, forest fires, lightning, and bacterial decay. That chemists can detect traces of these in the purest air should not be taken to mean that such traces do measurable harm. These substances are serious air pollutants only when the levels are much higher than in "pure" air.

If one takes a walk through the woods, he pollutes the air along his trail sufficiently so that a bloodhound can use his nose to follow him along that trail hours later. This is a tribute to the nose of the bloodhound, and does not suggest that we should never walk through the woods because by so doing we pollute the air. Pollutants, practically speaking, are objectionable only when quantitatively they are at harmful levels.

Similarly, typical "pure spring water" collected far from civilization contains dozens of minerals and other substances that would be highly objectionable in much larger quantities. We are biologically adapted to live with a small degree of pollution. Our environment, therefore, should not be expected to be perfect.

Our best foods—milk, meat, eggs, fish, cereals, fruits, vegetables, and nuts—also contain, even under the most favorable circumstances, detectable traces of such chemical elements as silver, titanium, barium, and strontium. All are highly toxic—*at higher levels*. These and other elements are picked up by plants and animals from the soil and water. If the soil contains an unusually large amount of some undesirable mineral, that mineral is absorbed by plants. Plants, too, have to be adapted to imperfect environments; hence, they contain traces that are passed on to the animals eating the plants. Sea water contains minute amounts of a wide assortment of minerals accumulated from the runoff of rivers. Marine organisms, therefore, including those we eat, do not find a perfect environment in sea water, and as a result, usually, contain traces of poisonous substances that could not be tolerated, by them or us, at higher levels.

We human beings, like other creatures, are so adapted that we can tolerate many kinds of poisonous minerals, provided the quantities present are very low. If we want to think of these minerals as pollutants, they are pollutants that we are biologically adapted to tolerate. Some of the "poisonous minerals" we find in foods in minute amounts may actually be beneficial. If there are essential trace elements that are yet to be recognized, they will be discovered in the list of poisonous chemicals found, for example, in sea water.

Our ability to adapt to imperfect environments and tolerate minute amounts of poisonous chemicals is further exemplified by the fact that many, if not all, natural foods contain traces of toxic substances (toxicants), many of which have been isolated chemically. These would be intolerable if the levels were high. Toxicants of this kind are present in such foods as potatoes and other vegetables, fruits, cereals, meats, nuts, cheese, and eggs. Depending on the kind of plant in which they originate, each toxicant is of a specific kind (often a glucoside or alkaloid). A strong reason for diversifying our food intake is to avoid getting too much of a single toxicant. We can tolerate much better minute amounts of various toxicants than we can higher concentrations of one. Among the plants which cannot safely be consumed, because they contain *intolerable* levels of toxicants are oleanders, tobacco, nightshade, castor beans, and poisonous mushrooms.

The presence of traces of various poisonous substances in our best air, water, and food should not blind us to the fact that pollution is all too frequently a real threat in modern life. It has been reliably estimated that, on the average, each adult consumes about three pounds of nonnutritive substances each year. This sounds less dramatic when it is realized that a person may consume nearly a ton of moist food per year and takes from the air in the course of a year approximately five hundred pounds of oxygen gas. Hundreds of unwanted chemical substances get into our food more or less accidentally. Among these are

141

insecticides and pesticides, and also the antibiotics fed to animals later slaughtered for food. Lead from leaded gasoline is another example of an accidental contaminant of water and food. Traces in the air from automobile exhaust find their way into plants and then into the animals or humans that eat the plants.

Among the nonnutritive substances that the Food and Drug Administration permits food manufacturers to put into foods are some mild preservatives like sodium benzoate and sodium propionate. These are regarded as harmless at the levels used and are very useful in preventing spoilage. Also permitted are certain substances like amyl acetate, which imparts a flavor like bananas and is similar chemically to natural fruit flavors. Certain supposedly nontoxic dyes are also permitted in some foods typically consumed in small amounts. Whether the Food and Drug Administration is too lenient in these matters may be debated—but the debate can be worthwhile only if the participants have an intelligent grasp of the whole pollution problem.

Among the food additives about which serious questions can be and have been raised are stilbestrol, an artificial, hormone-like substance that can be carcinogenic; artificial sweeteners (cyclamates and saccharin); and food dyes. Long ago, the use of "butter yellow," which is definitely carcinogenic, was prohibited. Monosodium glutamate has in recent years been found to be potentially harmful when used in relatively large amounts. This is the sodium salt of one of the amino acids we commonly derive in relatively large quantities from many proteins, especially plant proteins. Although its use to enhance the flavors of foods needs to be monitored, it is not essentially foreign to our bodies; hence, it does not belong in the same category with saccharin, food dyes, or stilbestrol.

The problem of pollution must be dealt with realistically and with some degree of consistency. There is no law of human nature, however, that can force the real people who make up our populations to be consistent. For example, some are fond of sound apples, yet decry the use of insecticides, which make sound apples possible. Some who cherish recorded music, beautiful man-made carpets, washable paints, and hundreds of other articles made from plastics are loath to accept responsibility for the chemical factories in which plastics are made. Many people buzzing around in automobiles would like to forget that every turn of an engine makes for some degree of pollution. They are matched, in inconsistency, by those who love lamb chops, yet think it is terrible to slaughter innocent lambs, and by those who want to build a world where everyone breeds freely, at the same time leaving room for everyone to live in a pleasant rural or suburban environment. All the problems and factors related to pollution must be balanced if we are to move in desirable directions.

Foreign substances entering our bodies are potentially harmful pollutants of our internal environments that may interfere with enzymic reactions and healthy metabolic processes. Foreign substances cannot act constructively, as do nutrients. At sufficiently high levels, any foreign substance can interfere with health.

Among the pollutants of our internal environments are the medicines we take. Probably the most widely used of these is aspirin. In the United States, it is used at the rate of about sixty tons per day. This is about one five-grain tablet per person per day, and would probably not cause serious trouble, provided it were contained in a time-released product and its consumption were evenly distributed in the adult population. Some people, however, take far more than their quota, and even deaths result, particularly among children, from overdoses. No one knows exactly why aspirin is physiologically effective, but by trial and error, it has been found to be at least a palliative for headaches and colds. It is one of the "pollutants" we deliberately put into our internal environments.

Because they are very effective medicines, antibiotics are used extensively. Because they interfere with metabolism in bacterial cells and impair the activities of bacteria, they also, inevitably, affect the metabolism of our own body cells to some extent, because of the strong resemblances among metabolic processes in all forms of life. For this reason, physicians do not as a rule advocate using antibiotics consistently and continually. In some cases, people can be made very ill by antibiotics, which are then dangerous pollutants.

People take many kinds of pills containing foreign substances: "pills to prevent sunburn," "pills to keep mosquitoes away," "pills to keep you awake," "pills to put you to sleep," "pills to prevent pregnancy," "pills to ease pain," "pills to make you high," "pills to help you quit smoking." All these are pollutants of our internal environment, and if they have any effect, good or bad, it is because they interfere with chemical processes taking place normally in the body. None of these is a constructive agent like nutritional minerals, amino acids, and vitamins which, in proper amounts, enhance healthy metabolism.

[Editor's note 1998: Partially hydrogenated fats contain unnatural kinds and amounts of fatty acids, and are now being recognized as harmful internal pollutants. They adversely affect the conversion of essential fatty acids into key hormone-like regulators such as prostaglandins, leukotrienes, and thromboxanes. As a result, they seem to increase risks for heart disease, high blood pressure, inflammatory diseases, and possibly many other conditions. Major sources of partially hydrogenated fats are solid margarine, vegetable shortening (used in a great many foods), and most peanut butter. Possible substitutes include liquid margarines, butter, liquid oils, and old-fashioned peanut butter.]

Other foreign agents that may contaminate our internal environment include caffeine, nicotine, alcohol, and drugs like LSD, amphetamines, marijuana, morphine, and heroin. Each of these acts in its own way; some are far more serious pollutants than others.

Caffeine is relatively harmless, and millions of people feel that they cannot get going in the morning without one or more cups of coffee. That caffeine is a drug, however, cannot be questioned; it is sold as such in tablets to keep people awake when they drive for long periods. The range of dosage necessary to stay awake varies widely from individual to individual.

How nicotine acts physiologically has been studied extensively, and many complexities and inconsistencies exist. In different metabolic situations such as exist in different individuals, its toxic effects may vary widely. In some individuals, heavy smoking causes dimness of vision and hemorrhagic areas in the retina. In others, it appears to cause severe circulatory disturbances, particularly in the legs (Buerger's disease), which may necessitate amputation. Statistical evidence indicates that some individuals have their lives shortened substantially (by several years) by the use of tobacco, but that those who survive smoking for a number of years are not much affected by continued smoking. Shortening of life is due, in considerable part, to heart impairment. Some individuals can stop smoking without difficulty; others are addicted, so that it is almost impossible for them to stop of their own volition. The smoking of cigarettes, which often involves inhaling the smoke, is a special hazard, particularly with respect to lung cancer. It should be noted, finally, that it cannot safely be asserted that the effects of tobacco are due solely to nicotine. In cigarette smoke, for example, there may be other harmful pollutants.

Alcohol has an unusual status. It is not completely foreign to the body, since small amounts are formed in metabolism. It can also be used as a fuel in the body. When introduced into our internal environment it can have many different effects, and in high concentrations may be highly toxic. Common signs of intoxication include vomiting, unsteady gait, slurred speech, hilarity, pugnacity, sleepiness, talkativeness, weeping, and double vision. The most serious toxic effect of alcohol, however, is impairment of the appetite mechanism in the brain to such an extent that the sight, taste, or smell of food is nauseating and nothing is attractive but alcohol itself. This undermines all nutrition and inevitably leads to disaster. Many people like alcohol and what it does to them so well that they accept the risks. For some, the pleasures of liquor consumption take precedence over almost everything else.

Marijuana smoking and the taking of drugs such as amphetamines and LSD have not been with us long enough for us to be completely certain of all their ill effects and just how serious these are. They are definitely pollutants of our internal environments. Each has its own dangers, and all interfere, in different ways and with different degrees of seriousness, with brain metabolism. All generate some desire on the part of the individuals using them to continue their use and gain the ephemeral "benefits."

Morphine and heroin are strongly addictive, and their use is, directly or indirectly, at the root of an enormous amount of crime. These are pollutants far more to be feared than the usual ones encountered in air, water, or food.

An important relationship between all internal pollutants and nutrition is this: superior nutrition, certainly in some cases and possibly in all, helps protect against the poisonous effects of pollutants. We have pointed out in another chapter that nutritional research has been inadequate to date and that, for this reason, there are many gaps in our knowledge. We now may add an additional gap to those already discussed. We do not know the extent to which good nutrition can protect people from pollutants. Recently, it has been found that animals living under smog conditions are healthier and live longer when their nutrition is improved. In other words, animals that are well fed can "thumb their noses" at minor air pollutants. How significant this observation is and how broadly the principle behind it applies is for the future to reveal. Certainly, the observation that good nutrition protects against some poisons is well founded.

XV

HOW TO CHOOSE
YOUR OWN NOURISHMENT

There is good news in this chapter for you, whether you are young, middle-aged, or elderly; whether you are in robust, mediocre, or poor health. There is also good news for pregnant women.

Hope for the future becomes brighter as we think of the potentialities of superior nutrition. Young people want to develop their bodies, minds, and personalities. Middle-aged and elderly people, if they are well, want to stay that way; if they are ill, they want relief. A pregnant woman wants to bring into the world a superior, well-developed baby. All these objectives can be realized only if nutrition is superior.

After the moment of conception, the dominant factor influencing our lives is the environment. Nutrition is a vital key to an environment of high quality. Aside from a suitable ambient temperature, water, and oxygen, nutrition is almost the complete story. Believing in the effectiveness of nutrition in our lives is like believing in the environment.

The minimum you can do if you are young, middle-aged, elderly, or a pregnant woman is to concentrate on good, wholesome foods and to exercise enough so that the nutrients are adequately distributed every day. (The expression "good, wholesome food," by the way, should not be taken to suggest that such food must be dull or unappetizing. Attractiveness is certainly important.)

Which are the good, wholesome foods? How can they be spotted and evaluated? In what ways are foods likely to lack good quality? As a help in answer-

149

ing these questions, my colleague, Dr. Donald R. Davis, and I have devised a series of charts, each representing a particular food. Before you look at them, let me explain briefly why they are constructed as they are and how they are to be interpreted.

We have already discussed in Chapter V that there are some parts of the total environment that we usually do not have to be much concerned about. However, the crucial thing which cannot be neglected is the adequate presence in our food of all the *growth and maintenance chemicals*. If any of these is inadequately supplied, all the cells in our bodies suffer. The quality of the environment we furnish our hearts, kidneys, muscles, brains, etc., determines how well these structures function.

If our charts depicting individual foods and food mixtures are to be useful, they must tell something about how well these foods supply the growth and maintenance chemicals. These vital nutrients are the a b c's of scientific nutrition and may be thought of as the "nutritional alphabet." The quality of a food cannot be judged unless we can recognize its ability to furnish the "alphabet items."

All good, wholesome foods furnish calories balanced by significant amounts of the growth and maintenance chemicals. In these charts we have postulated a daily food intake of 2,500 calories, accompanied by the required amounts of all the growth and maintenance chemicals (see Table 1, page 28). (The more energy-containing food we consume, the more growth and maintenance chemicals we need.) The diagrams tell of the ability of each food depicted to perform essential nutritional functions. Each diagram, thus, gives a picture of the *trophic* value of a food—its ability to supply the essentials above and beyond energy or calories. Each one shows, in essence, what kinds and amounts of growth and maintenance chemicals a person could obtain from a particular food if he were to satisfy an average day's energy requirement by eating *that food alone*. The object is *not* to encourage anyone to do this, but rather to provide easy-to-understand comparisons between various foods. I am especially grateful to Dr. Davis for supervising the collection and computer analysis of the extensive data represented by the diagrams.

In each of these cartwheel-type diagrams, we have forty-two dotted lines radiating from a center. Beginning at about the three o'clock position on each diagram, these lines represent the growth and maintenance chemicals, as follows:

Amino Acids:	Histidine (His), Isoleucine (Isol), Leucine (Leu), Lysine (Lys), Methionine (Met), Phenylalanine (Phe), Threonine (Thr), Tryptophan (Try), Valine (Val).
Vitamins*:	Vitamin A (A), Biotin (Bio), Vitamin B_6 (B_6), Vitamin B_{12} (B_{12}), Vitamin C (C), Vitamin D (D), Vitamin E (E), Folic acid (Fol), Vitamin K (K), Niacin (Nia), Pantothenic acid (Pan), Riboflavin (Ribo), Thiamin (Thia).
Major Minerals:	Calcium (Ca), Chloride (Cl), Potassium (K), Magnesium (Mg), Sodium (Na), Phosphate PO_4).
Trace Minerals:	Cobalt (Co), Chromium (Cr), Copper (Cu), Fluorine (F), Iron (Fe), Iodine (I), Manganese (Mn), Molybdenum (Mo), Selenium (Se), Zinc (Zn).
Other:	Choline (Cho), Fiber, Linoleic acid (Lin), Omega-3 fatty acids (Omg3).

151

In diagramming each of the forty different foods, we have drawn on top of the radiating dotted lines heavy black lines whose lengths indicate the amounts of the various nutritional items contained in a food. These amounts are not expressed in terms of milligrams or grams but, rather, in terms of how well they fill estimated adult needs. If a particular heavy black line extends from the center halfway to the inner circle, this means that the maintenance item represented is half enough; if another heavy black line extends out past the inner circle, it means that more than enough is supplied to meet the estimated daily adult needs.

Consider, for example, figure 14, representing a hypothetical food containing the estimated daily adult needs for all the growth and maintenance chemicals. The *quality* of this hypothetical food is such that a *quantity* of it providing 2,500 calories of energy would also contain exactly the estimated daily adult requirement of all the growth and maintenance chemicals (see table 1, page 28). A lesser or greater amount of this hypothetical food would yield either less or more energy, plus a proportionate amount of the nutritional essentials. This matching of energy and the estimated amounts of the nutritional essentials has been indicated by drawing heavy black lines on

*The nomenclature of vitamins often seems confusing. Originally, when there were thought to be very few vitamins, letters of the alphabet were used in naming them. When "vitamin B" turned out to be a number of different vitamins, subscript numerals were used (B_1, B_2). This nomenclature has been retained in some cases for complex historical reasons. More recently, however, biochemists have been inclined to use the chemical names of the substances involved (thiamin, riboflavin, niacinamide, pantothenic acid, biotin, folic acid) rather than numerical subscripts. The members of the B family of vitamins are completely distinct entities, not parts of "vitamin B."

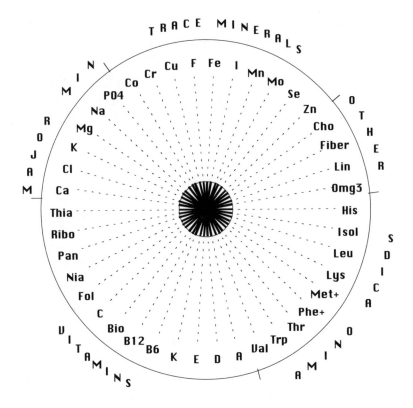

Figure 14. **Hypothetical food** (containing the estimated adult needs of each maintenance chemical).

top of all of the forty-two dotted lines, beginning at the center and going out to the inner circle. This hypothetical food would be an ideal food for adults *if* all adults were about the same and *if* the "estimated needs" were all accurately assessed.

Next, let us consider figure 15. Here, all the dotted lines are empty; that is, no heavy black lines have been drawn. This means that no maintenance chemicals are present. This diagram represents such "foods" as sugar, glucose (dextrose), corn syrup, alcohol, starch (dextrine), and saturated fat, none of which contains substantial amounts of any of the growth and maintenance chemicals. (They yield only energy—no balancing amounts of essential nutrients.) Again, this diagram tells of *quality* (or, rather, lack of it) and applies to any *quantity* of these "foods," as long as the storage supply of nutritional essentials in the body holds out.

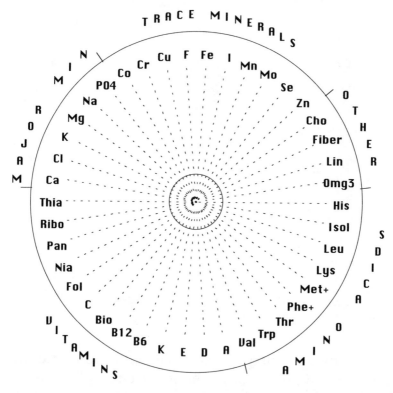

Figure 15. **"Foods" containing no maintenance chemicals (sugar, glucose, alcohol, starch, saturated fat).** 1.4 pounds or 650 grams of sugar yield 2,500 calories, and this amount at 40 cents a pound would cost 60 cents. 2 pounds or 890 grams of glucose syrup yield 2,500 calories. This amount at $1.50 a pound would cost $2.90. About 1.05 liters of whiskey yield 2,500 calories. This amount at $8.00 per liter would cost $8.50. 1.5 pounds or 660 grams of starch yield 2,500 calories. This amount at $1.00 per pound would cost $1.50. 10 ounces or 290 grams of saturated fat yield 2,500 calories. This amount at 80 cents per pound would cost 50 cents.

The purpose of charts like figures 14, 15, and the succeeding ones (figures 16 to 54) is to help you to understand the nature of "good, wholesome food" so that you will be better able to choose your own nourishment intelligently. Most of the foods diagrammed—grains, eggs, milk, meats, fish, oysters, cheeses, beans, potatoes, numerous vegetables, fruits, melons, mushrooms, and peanuts—are "good, wholesome foods," as evidenced by the fact that each furnishes, besides energy, a substantial assortment of most of the growth and maintenance chemicals.

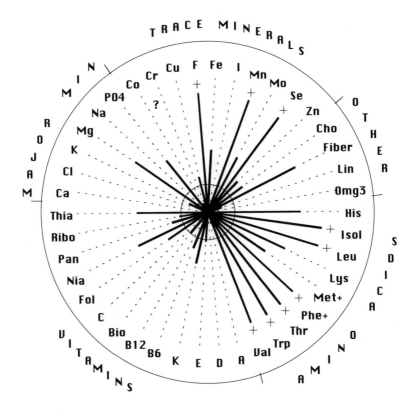

Figure 16. **Wheat.** 1.7 pounds or 760 grams yield 2,500 calories. This amount at 40 cents per pound would cost 65 cents.

There are many other good, wholesome foods besides those diagrammed. The enormous variety of these is a great advantage because foods that are relatively weak in certain respects can be supplemented by others that are relatively richer sources of specific growth and maintenance chemicals. Also, tastes differ—and this means that many people will want to substitute other foods for those they do not enjoy. Notice that many of the foods diagrammed contribute far *more* than the estimated daily requirements of certain maintenance chemicals. In explain-

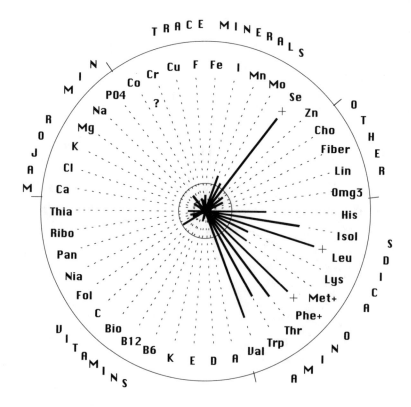

Figure 17. **White flour.** 1.5 pounds or 690 grams yield 2,500 calories. This amount at 25 cents per pound would cost 40 cents.

ing this, several considerations may be of assistance. First, the estimated (average) needs (for maximum good health) may actually be too low. Second, the needs of small children, older children, and pregnant women are certainly often far higher than those of "average" adults. (This may also be true of the elderly.) Third, the needs of some individuals are far above average, and it appears that nature takes into account real people such as these, whose needs would not be met, for example, by the hypothetical food represented in the first diagram. Fourth, almost no

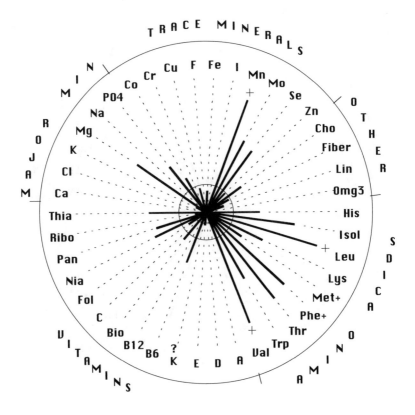

Figure 18. **Rice, grain (brown).** 1.5 pounds or 680 grams yield 2,500 calories. This amount at 70 cents per pound would cost $1.05

food is completely adequate with regard to all nutrients, and richer sources are needed to compensate for
the poorer sources. Fifth, we are adapted, biologically,
to consume wholesome foods such as those diagrammed.

To depict the content of each food charted, we
have had to rely on the best information available
concerning that food's composition. Another limita-
tion is that different samples of the same food are not
usually equal in composition. In specific instances,
the variation among samples is large. Owing to this

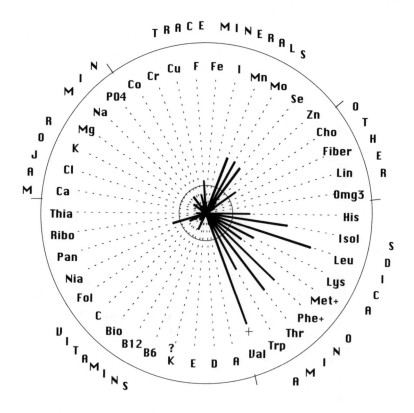

Figure 19. **Rice, white (milled).** 1.5 pounds or 690 grams yield
2,500 calories. This amount at 60 cents per pound would cost 90
cents.

uncertainty and uncertainties related to human requirements, these diagrams give information about
the *quality* of the specific foods, but they are only
approximations *quantitatively*.

Some gaps exist in the available information. We
have left a question mark in the appropriate space
when a food has not been analyzed for a specific
maintenance chemical; we have left the appropriate
dotted line unchanged when analysis has not revealed the presence of the item. Data are not complete, adequate, or clear for items such as vitamin B_{12},

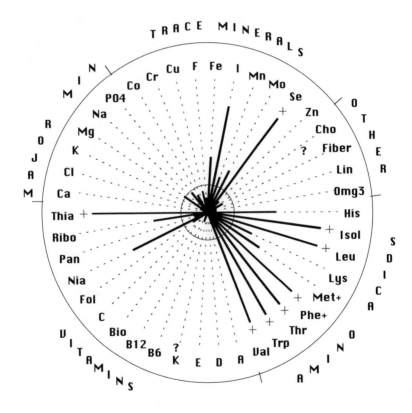

Figure 20. **Macaroni.** 1.5 pounds or 670 grams yield 2,500
calories. This amount at $1.00 per pound would cost $1.50.

vitamin D, vitamin K, linoleic acid, and some trace minerals. Vitamin B_{12}, believed to be absent from plant tissues, does not appear in the charts depicting plant foods. There may be traces of vitamin B_{12}, however, and the fact that bacteria in the digestive tract may produce it complicates the situation further. Vitamin D is not known to be present in most foods, but relatively rich sources exist and this vitamin is produced by the action of sunlight. Therefore, there has been little concern for traces of vitamin D that may be in foods that are not good sources. The

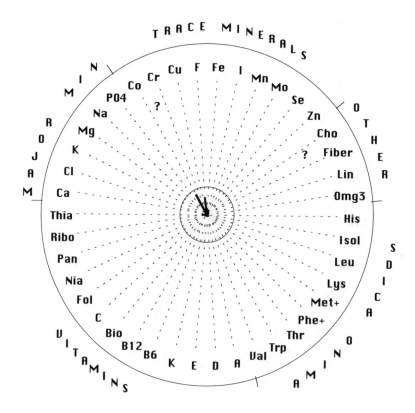

Figure 21. **Honey.** 1.8 pounds or 820 grams yield 2,500 calories. This amount at $2.00 per pound would cost $3.60.

small amounts of vitamin K that may be present in various foods receive little attention because this vitamin is produced by intestinal bacteria. Linoleic acid is one of the fatty acids, and scientists have not adequately explored its presence in foods of low fat content. To complicate matters, the estimated needs for these and some other nutrients are subject to large uncertainties.

The "equal calorie" method of depicting foods is one of the many ways of presenting information about foods. We regard it as valuable and instructive be-

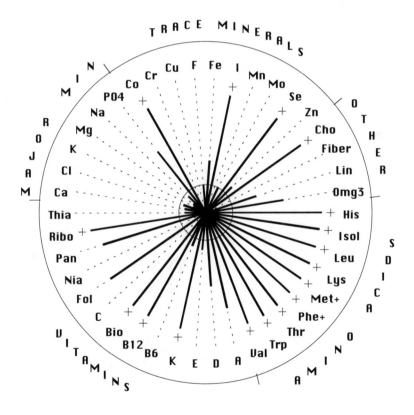

Figure 22. **Eggs.** 33 eggs (large) yield 2,500 calories. This amount at $1.00 per dozen would cost $2.80.

cause it reveals food quality and takes into account the important fact that the more calories one consumes, the more maintenance chemicals one needs. As nutritional science develops further, charts of this kind will improve in accuracy. In a true sense, our charts are preliminary in nature. A potential weakness is that the "nutritional alphabet" may be incomplete; discovery and recognition, in the future, of additional nutrients is probable.

The plus marks at the ends of the heavy black lines in many of the charts signify that the black line

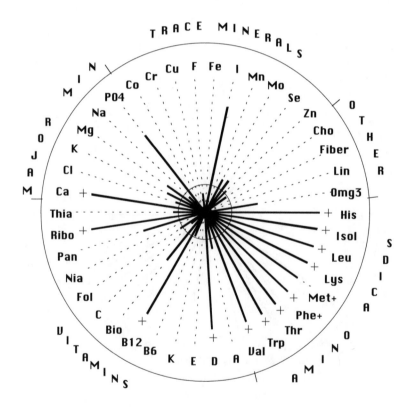

Figure 23. **Milk (whole).** 1.05 gallons or 4.0 liters yield 2,500 calories. This amount at $2.00 per gallon would cost $2.10.

would extend still further but for lack of space. Below the charts for the various foods, we list the approximate amounts (in common units and in grams or kilograms) of the food required to furnish 2,500 calories—about one day's supply of energy. We do not suggest, as I have already explained, that anyone will get an entire day's energy supply from any one food (wide diversification is urgently recommended), but the estimates are nevertheless useful for comparison. The estimated cost of 2,500 calories of each food is also given for purposes of comparison. Although these

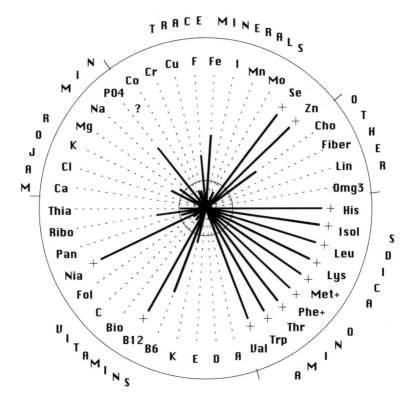

Figure 24. **Beef.** 5.4 pounds or 2.4 kilograms (allowing for 30% waste) yield 2,500 calories. This amount at $3.00 per pound would cost $16.

figures are only approximations, for reasons already mentioned, the wide divergences among different types of food should be noted.

The charts certainly should not convey the idea that nutrition is simple or that they tell the whole story. Some of the complications that concern experts involve the fact that one's need for a maintenance chemical often depends on the supply of other nutrients. For example, the need for methionine is decreased by significant quantities of cystine and/or an abundant supply of choline; in turn, the methionine

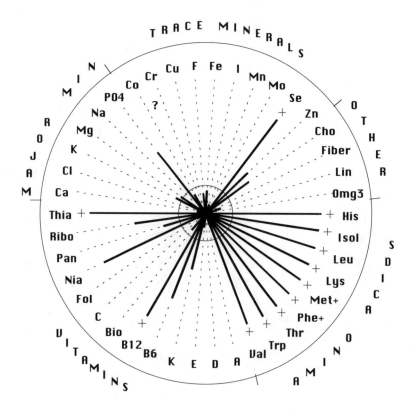

Figure 25. **Pork.** 5.5 pounds or 2.5 kilograms (allowing for 30% waste) yield 2,500 calories. This amount at $2.50 per pound would cost $14.

supply influences the choline requirements. Similarly, the presence of tyrosine decreases the need for phenylalanine. Also, the supply of vitamin B_{12} influences the need for folic acid, and vice versa. There are many potential balances and imbalances between specific minerals. Many interrelationships among nutrients exist that cannot be shown on the charts.

Our diagrams also do not depict certain other factors related to the foods we eat. Sometimes, maintenance chemicals are present in foods but are not fully available. For example, certain individuals may

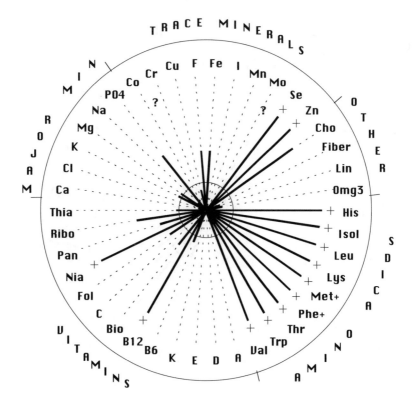

Figure 26. **Lamb.** 7.1 pounds or 3.2 kilograms (allowing for 40% waste) yield 2,500 calories. This amount at $3.00 per pound would cost $21.30.

digest proteins with difficulty and, thus, fail to receive the full complement of amino acids present in a food. Also, oxalic acid or phytic acid, sometimes present in foods, can cause calcium (and some other minerals) to become insoluble and, thus, not fully useful.

In addition, our charts do not depict how foods might differ in value depending on the method of preparation. The values we have given in general apply to the foods at purchase. Cooking with large amounts of water may leach out some of the minerals and other water-soluble nutrients; cooking or drying

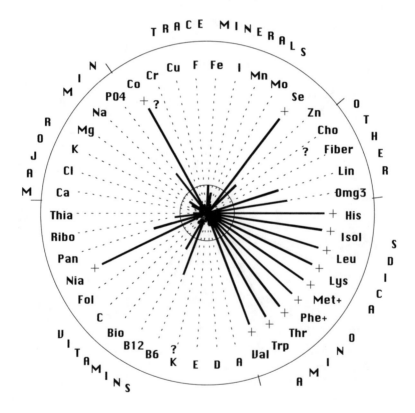

Figure 27. **Chicken.** 9.6 pounds or 4.4 kilograms (allowing for 50% waste) yield 2,500 calories. This amount at $1.00 per pound would cost $9.60.

in the presence of air causes the destruction of vitamin C (ascorbic acid).

Finally, our diagrams do not show the presence or absence of the small amounts of harmful substances that foods often contain. As long as these toxicants remain at low levels of concentration, the body can prevent their toxic effects. One of the strong arguments for diversifying our foods is that, by doing so, we avoid too high a concentration of any one toxicant. Human beings can tolerate minute amounts of several toxicants, but a relatively high concentration of

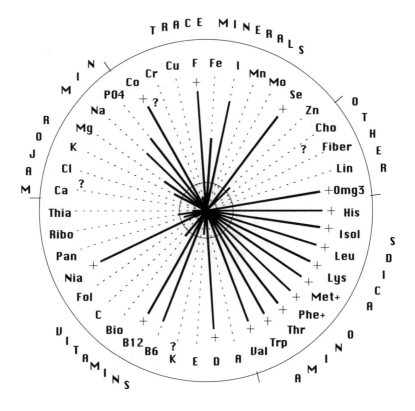

Figure 28. **Fish (tuna, canned in water, salted).** 4.8 pounds or 2.2 kilograms (15 six-ounce cans, allowing for 15% liquid) yield 2,500 calories. This amount at $1.50 per pound would cost $7.10.

any one may cause trouble. Just as our atmospheric environment is imperfect, so also is our food environment. One of the ways it is imperfect is that foods often contain small amounts of substances that can be very toxic. The pharmacist marks oxalic acid with skull and crossbones. In sufficient amounts, it is highly toxic. Yet many plant foods contain oxalic acid (oxalis leaves and spinach are notable examples). At low levels, its potential bad effect is limited to making a certain amount of calcium unavailable. The milling of wheat (see figures 16 and 17) causes a loss in its

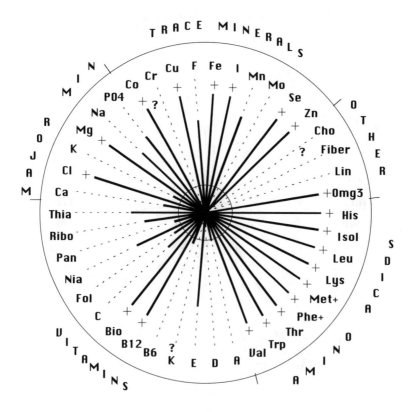

Figure 29. **Oysters.** 9.3 pounds or 4.2 kilograms yield 2,500 calories. This amount at $6.00 per pound would cost $56.

nutritional quality—minor losses in amino acids, and major losses in minerals and vitamins. The average loss for all the maintenance chemicals is over 50 percent. The milling of rice has about the same effect on the nutritional quality of this grain. Such losses may be very serious because foods derived from these grains often contribute a large percentage of the food energy which individuals get.

The minimum we should do to guard our nutrition and the inner environment of all our body cells and tissues is to diversify our food choices, concen-

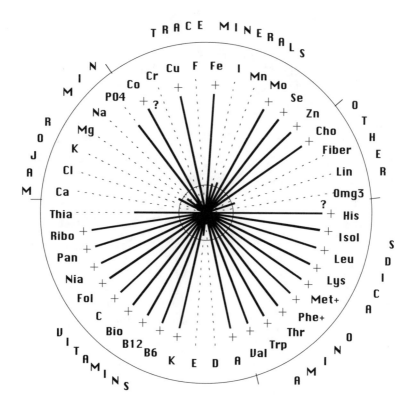

Figure 30. **Liver.** 3.9 pounds or 1.7 kilograms yield 2,500 calories. This amount at $1.30 per pound would cost $5.00.

trate on wholesome foods, and exercise adequately so that the nutrients will reach the cells that need them continuously. When selecting from the large number of wholesome foods, we should consider these factors: (1) *foods chosen should be liked*; (2) *their cost should not be prohibitive; and* (3) *they should be readily and agreeably accepted by our bodies.* When wholesome foods meet these requirements, they can be consumed in relatively large quantities. If this principle were generally followed, human nutrition would be immeasurably improved.

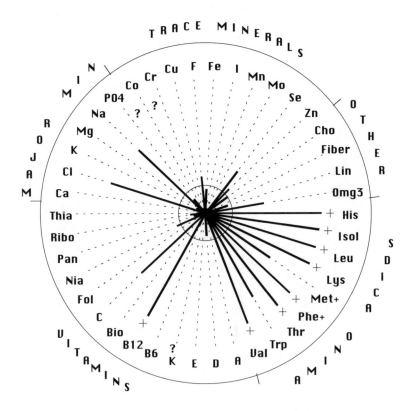

Figure 31. **Frankfurters (all meat).** 1.7 pounds or 780 grams yield 2,500 calories. This amount at $2.50 per pound would cost $4.30.

These "good, wholesome foods" are available in nature for the nourishment not only of human beings but of all members of the animal kingdom, from the largest to the most microscopic. They are, in the absence of human intervention, virtually the only foods available to animals. They are capable of promoting excellent development and health.

Because of what I have referred to as the "smarty pants" attitude of human beings when they think cooperation with nature is unnecessary, we have available many other "foods" to tempt us which, as

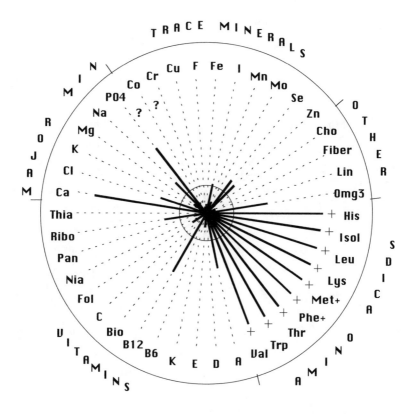

Figure 32. **Cheese (cheddar).** 1.4 pounds or 620 grams yield 2,500 calories. This amount at $3.50 per pound would cost $4.80.

foods, are not wholesome at all. Conspicuous examples are sugar, glucose, starch, alcohol, and refined, saturated fat. All are energy sources, but the more meticulous we are about our nutrition, the more we will avoid relying on these as such. We will seek, instead, to obtain our energy from sources which also furnish the essentials for good health.

Figures 16 to 19 show how whole grain foods have been converted into products far less wholesome. Partial restorations to correct the previous milling errors are included in these diagrams. The damage

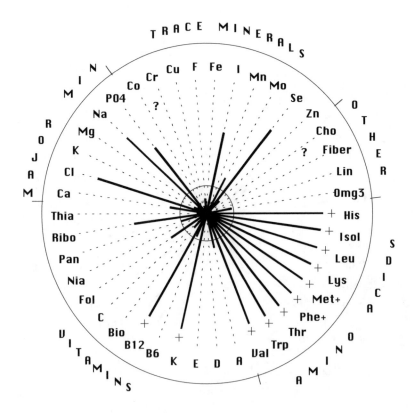

Figure 33. **Cottage cheese.** 5.4 pounds or 2.4 kilograms yield 2,500 calories. This amount at $1.70 per pound would cost $9.10.

done to our nutrition by the use of white flour and white rice is considerable, because these products often furnish a large part of an individual's food energy, particularly (but not solely) in the case of people who cannot afford meats and other wholesome, but expensive, foods. Many cereal-containing products, for example, contain white flour, and even those breads ostensibly made from whole grain nevertheless contain a substantial amount of white flour. Impairment of food quality by the use of white flour is augmented by the extensive use of sugar, syrup, and

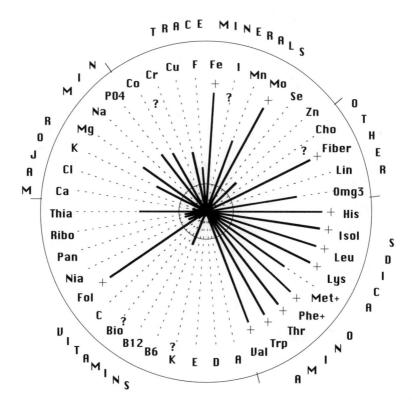

Figure 34. **Beans (dry).** 1.6 pounds or 740 grams yield 2,500 calories. This amount at 60 cents per pound would cost 95 cents.

shortening, not only in a great variety of bakery goods but also in other cookery. The damage done to our diets by extensive use of sugar, white flour, and white rice is further augmented, often to an alarming degree, by extensive use of alcohol. Those who ignore common sense cooperation with nature by habitually taking one drink after another at frequent intervals are building poor nutrition and a poor internal environment almost as effectively as if they were trying to accomplish this dire purpose.

A perusal of the charts should dispel certain very

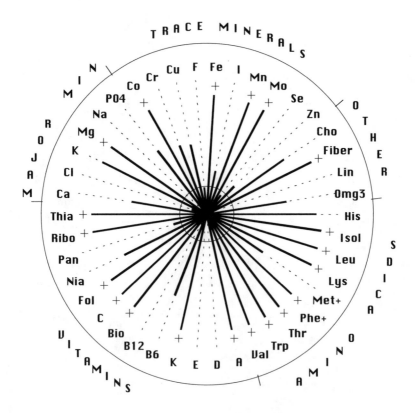

Figure 35. **String beans.** 20 pounds or 9.2 kilograms (allowing for 12% waste) yield 2,500 calories. This amount at $1.00 per pound would cost $20.

common oversimplifications exemplified by such statements as "Milk furnishes calcium," "Carrots give us vitamin A," "Red meat furnishes iron," and "Oranges give us vitamin C." Although these statements are literally true, they tell such a small fraction of the whole truth that they are misleading. Every one of the wholesome foods just mentioned furnishes substantial amounts of at least 90 percent of the growth and maintenance chemicals. Similarly, I think it may be surprising to many nutritionists to learn that such foods as lettuce, cabbage, oysters, and mushrooms

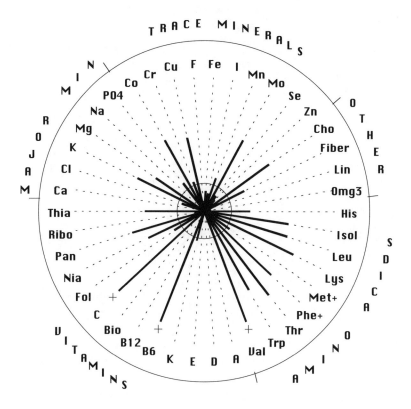

Figure 36. **Potatoes.** 9.3 pounds or 4.2 kilograms (allowing for 25% peelings and waste) yield 2,500 calories. This amount at 40 cents per pound would cost $3.70.

175

are excellent sources (on an equal calorie basis) of
most of the nutritional essentials, including the essential amino acids.

These facts about good nourishing foods reinforce
three important thoughts about nutrition that I have
voiced before. First, there is a tremendous unity in all
of nature. We human beings certainly do not greatly
resemble lettuce plants; yet, when we examine lettuce plants for the presence of our growth and maintenance chemicals, we find that most of them are
present—and in appropriate amounts. Neither let-

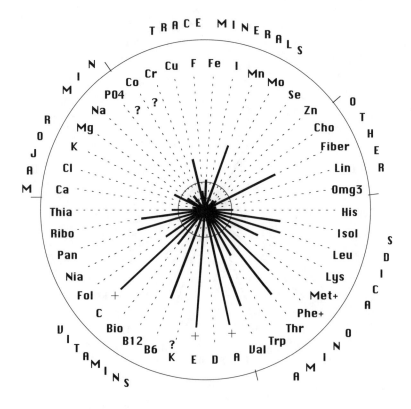

Figure 37. **Sweet potatoes.** 7.3 pounds or 3.3 kilograms
(allowing for 30% peelings and waste) yield 2,500 calories. This
amount at 70 cents per pound would cost $5.10.

tuce plants nor human beings can live without such chemicals as calcium, phosphate, zinc, copper, and molybdenum. Second, metabolism requires the presence of a large number of different chemical entities. If one link in the essential chain is missing, metabolism fails utterly. Nutrition must supply *every* link in the chain. Third, because of the large number of nutrients involved and the way foods differ in quality, it becomes obvious that diets will always vary in quality and can be altered in many ways by making different food choices. If all the available foods are

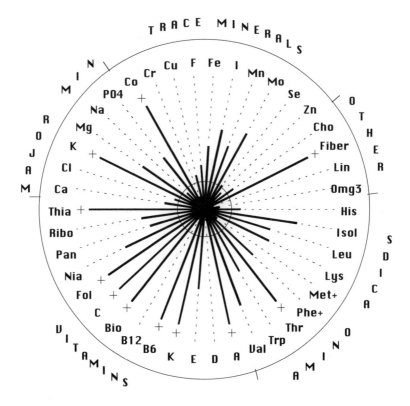

Figure 38. **Carrots.** 14.4 pounds or 6.5 kilograms (allowing for 10% waste) yield 2,500 calories. This amount at 70 cents per pound would cost $10.

considered, including those that mainly yield calories, it is possible to have diets of greatly varying quality—very poor, poor, mediocre, good, and excellent.

It should be noted, on the basis of the information accompanying the diagrams, that some foods—particularly watery vegetables and fruits—are not suitable as sources of large proportions of our food energy. To "keep going" on such foods alone, one would have to consume very large amounts of them. They cannot, therefore, make up a large percentage of one's diet.

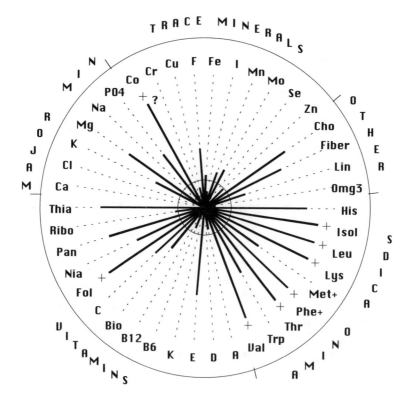

Figure 39. **Sweet corn (off the cob).** 6.4 pounds or 2.9 kilograms yield 2,500 calories. This amount at $1.10 per pound would cost $8.00.

Other foods, like oysters and mushrooms, are too expensive to constitute a major part of a person's diet. Nothing revealed in these charts should be interpreted as cancelling out the desirable use of common sense in the selection of foods.

The chart for eggs (figure 22) calls attention to the fact that eggs are an excellent source of amino acids and many other nutrients. This food has one conspicuous lack—vitamin C. As I have noted earlier, most animals make vitamin C internally and do not need to receive it from the food environment. Humans, monkeys, and guinea pigs, however, cannot produce it

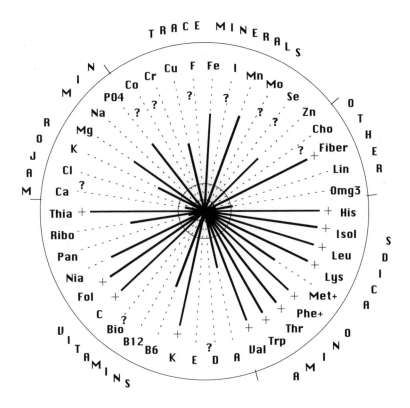

Figure 40. **Green peas.** 7.2 pounds or 3.2 kilograms yield 2,500 calories. This amount at $1.00 per pound would cost $7.20.

internally and require it in their diets. For young rats, cooked egg alone is almost a perfect diet. For them, the lack of vitamin C doesn't matter. Uncooked egg is a different story; it contains avidin (destroyed by cooking), a protein that combines with biotin furnished by the egg in such a way as to render it useless. On raw egg, rats are biotin deficient.

Egg is very low in niacinamide, one of the essential B vitamins. It is interesting, however, that eggs are very rich in the amino acid tryptophan, high levels of which can be made into niacinamide in the body.

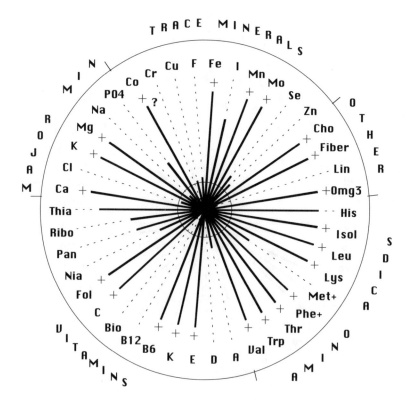

Figure 41. **Cabbage.** 27.5 pounds or 12.5 kilograms (allowing for 20% waste) yield 2,500 calories. This amount at 40 cents per pound would cost $11.

Biologically, egg is everything necessary to build a complete baby chick. Incidentally, a baby chick, when hatched, has a good supply of vitamin C, manufactured internally during development.

Barring the existence of allergy to egg protein, eggs are an extremely valuable human food. Although they contain substantial amounts of cholesterol, it is very doubtful, in my opinion, if this is, generally speaking, a fault. Eggs also contain high amounts of lecithin, which helps protect against the deposit of cholesterol in arteries. There are still many unan-

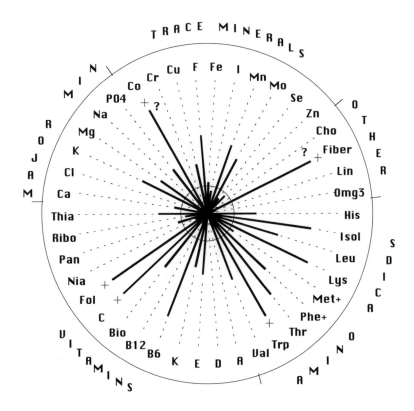

Figure 42. **Onions.** 16 pounds or 7.3 kilograms (allowing for 10% waste) yield 2,500 calories. This amount at 50 cents per pound would cost $8.10.

swered questions concerning cholesterol.

Milk, represented in figure 23, is also an excellent source of amino acids and many other nutrients. Its conspicuous deficiencies are its low iron, copper, and chromium contents. Young animals for which milk is nature's food have iron and other trace minerals in storage at birth. Hence, they do not have to receive these nutrients during the early stages of growth. Young rats, for example, can thrive on milk alone and do not need extra iron until they have almost reached sexual maturity. The presence of very high levels of

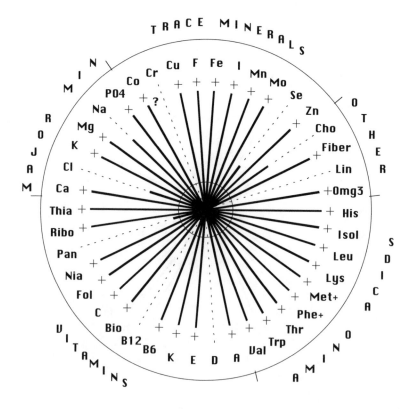

Figure 43. **Spinach.** 23 pounds or 10.4 kilograms of spinach yield 2,500 calories. This amount at $1.30 per pound would cost $30.

the essential amino acids in milk suggests that the amino acid needs of children and young adults are probably high. Actually, analyses show that milk often furnishes ten or even fifteen times the amount of amino acids needed by the hypothetical adult. Nature probably has good reason for furnishing these high amounts in the food it has designed for the young. Either *all* young animals need *all* the amino acids at high levels, or extra high amounts are furnished to fill the needs of individual animals with unusually high requirements. In any case, the facts

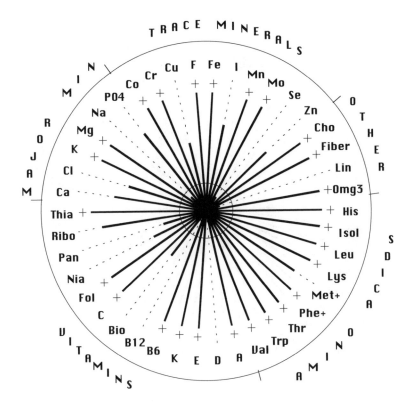

Figure 44. **Lettuce.** 45 pounds or 20 kilograms (allowing for 5% waste) yield 2,500 calories. This amount at 70 cents per pound would cost $31.

suggest strongly that children and young adults need far more of the amino acids (and probably other nutrients) than does the hypothetical adult. This does not preclude the conclusion that some adults may also benefit from levels much higher than the requirements of the hypothetical adult.

For the most part, the charts representing the other single foods speak for themselves; it would take far too much space to discuss each food individually. Our knowledge about quantitative needs for many of the nutrients is, as I have said, uncertain, and nutri-

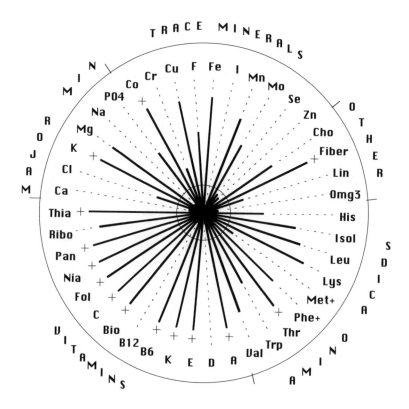

Figure 45. **Tomatoes.** 29 pounds or 13 kilograms (allowing for 10% waste) yield 2,500 calories. This amount at $1.30 per pound would cost $37.

tional science has not advanced to the point at which we can evaluate foods with complete satisfaction.

Care is advised in drawing conclusions from the charts about those nutrients about which we know the least, such as cobalt, chromium, fluorine, manganese, molybdenum, selenium, vitamin D, vitamin E, choline, and linoleic acid. Foods do not deserve a strong demerit if they are low in nutrients, such as biotin and vitamin K, known to be produced by intestinal bacteria. The data with respect to a number of nutrients are suggestive rather than conclusive. You

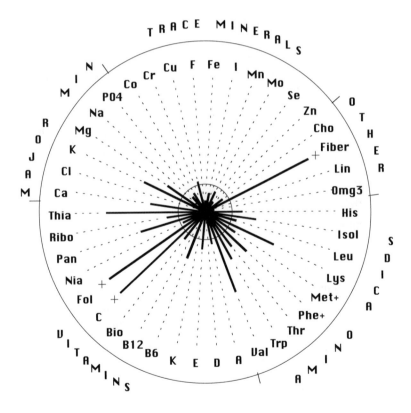

Figure 46. **Oranges.** 16 pounds or 7.3 kilograms (allowing for 25% waste) yield 2,500 calories. This amount at 60 cents per pound would cost $9.60.

will also note that many foods appear to be deficient in chloride and sodium. It is not accidental that sodium chloride (ordinary salt) is commonly on the dining table. Because many foods are deficient in iodine (depending in part on where they are grown), there is justification for supplementing our diets with iodized salt.

Meats (including fish) are excellent sources of the essential amino acids and vitamin B_{12}, but tend to be low in calcium and incomplete in other ways. Pork is an unusually good source of thiamin.

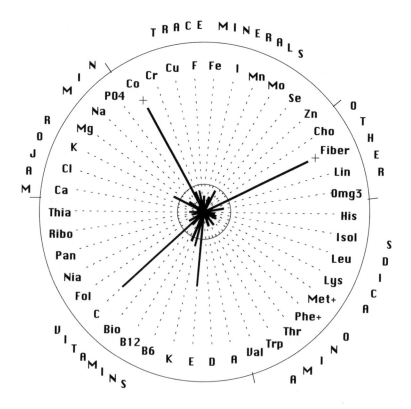

Figure 47. **Apples.** 10 pounds or 4.6 kilograms (allowing for 8% waste) yield 2,500 calories. This amount at $1.00 per pound would cost $10.

In general, vegetables tend to be less well supplied with essential amino acids and to lack vitamin B_{12}, but they are sometimes good sources of calcium. Methionine is often conspicuously more deficient in vegetables than most of the other essential amino acids. It is difficult to generalize about vegetables because there is great diversity among them. Lettuce is a remarkably well rounded food; aside from being somewhat deficient in methionine and lacking in vitamin B_{12}, it seems to supply most nutrients in abundance. Cabbage resembles it; it is relatively

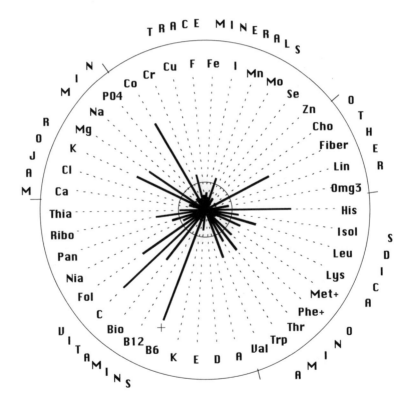

Figure 48. **Bananas.** 9.2 pounds or 4.2 kilograms (allowing for 35% waste) yield 2,500 calories. This amount at 50 cents per pound would cost $4.60.

deficient in both methionine and phenylalanine and lacks vitamin B_{12}. An important drawback of these foods, as we have seen, is that it takes so much of them to furnish adequate calories. Cabbage has the added disadvantage of containing goiter-producing agents that may affect persons who consume large amounts. (As we saw in Chapter XIV, many natural foods contain small amounts of harmful substances.)

Consideration of these diagrams leads us to appreciate that maintenance chemicals and calories go together in the whole of nature. When a proper bal-

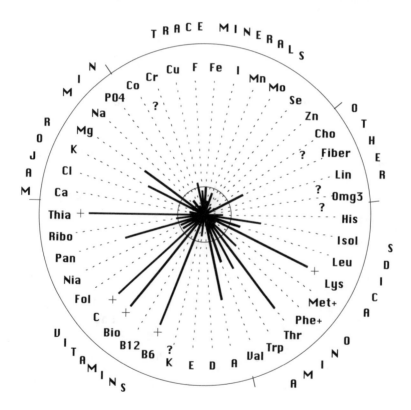

Figure 49. **Watermelon.** 33 pounds or 15 kilograms (allowing for 50% waste) yield 2,500 calories. This amount at 25 cents per pound (in season) would cost $8.30.

ance exists between the calories on one hand and the maintenance chemicals on the other, a good food results. A food that is appropriate for one species of animals is likely to be basically good for other animals. A diet that is good for a rat, for example, is a relatively good diet for a guinea pig, monkey, or human if we add vitamin C. Such a diet will be basically good for chickens if we assure the adequate presence of glycine. (This amino acid is nutritionally essential for chickens but not for mammals.)

We have data for high quality commercial dog

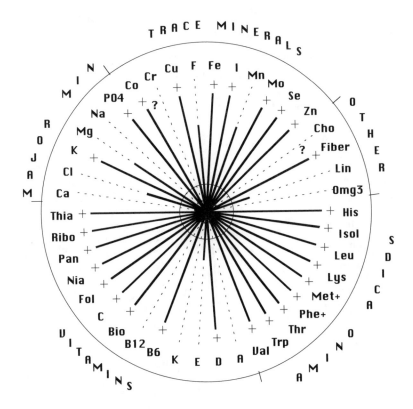

Figure 50. **Mushrooms.** 23 pounds or 10 kilograms (allowing for 3% waste) yield 2,500 calories. This amount at $3.50 per pound would cost $79.

189

food, rat food, and monkey food. Figure 52 shows the contents of dog food. Commercial foods for other animals show a strong resemblance to dog food. Many of these animal foods are of high nutritional quality. They have to be, to compete. Of course, different species benefit from different food mixtures. Basically, however, there is always a balance between calories and many of the same maintenance items. Even the diet of as distant a relative as an insect larva, if diagrammed, would show many marked resemblances to mammalian foods. Our charts are,

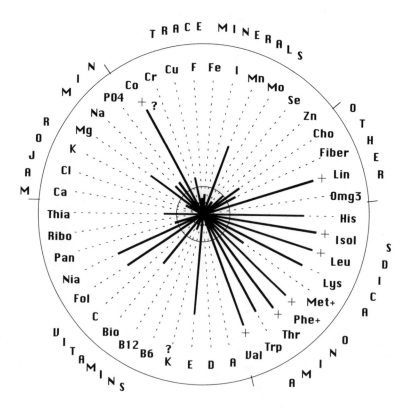

Figure 51. **Peanuts.** 15 ounces or 430 grams yield 2,500 calories. This amount at $2.50 per pound would cost $2.35.

therefore, of wide significance.

Let us now consider figure 53: the "average" American diet. It is average in the sense that my colleague, Dr. Davis, formulated it from Department of Agriculture tables showing American food consumption and calculated the data on the basis of appropriate amounts of the foods actually consumed. This is a very diversified diet and, in this respect, superior to that of a typical individual citizen since he does not, of course, consume as wide a variety of foods as is represented by this diagram.

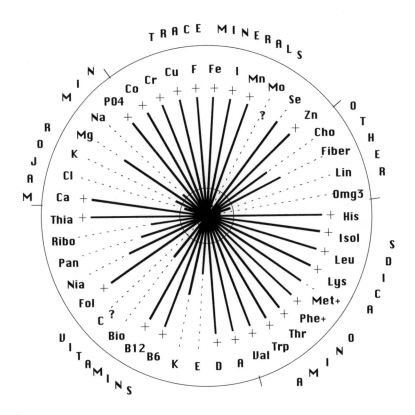

Figure 52. **Commercial dog food.** 1.5 pounds or 680 grams yield 2,500 calories. This amount at 52 cents per pound would cost 78 cents.

Note that this diverse diet contains some of every nutrient but that it is low (two-thirds or less of the estimate) with respect to nine items. If we compare figures 52 and 53, we see that dog food resembles a "perfect" food far more closely than does the "average" American diet, even though this represents something superior to what typical Americans actually consume. This is, or should be, an alarming observation, especially when we recognize that something like the "average" American diet, or even something inferior to it, is consumed by children, whose require-

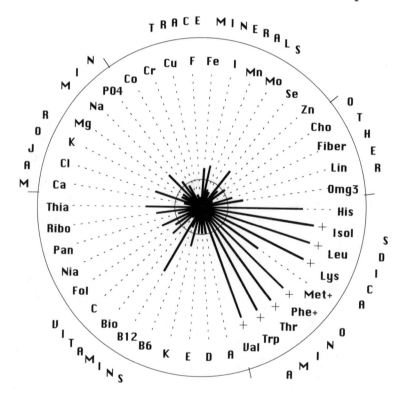

Figure 53. **"Average" American diet.** This is calculated on the basis of total American food consumption figures from the U.S. Department of Agriculture. It does not accurately represent the food consumed by any individual. The complete assortment is more diversified than that consumed by individual people.

ments are far more exacting than those of adults.

Figure 54 shows the results of the analysis of the foods actually consumed by a particular individual (Dr. Davis) over a three-month period. He selected commonly available foods during this time but avoided those with added sugar and those, such as bread and pastry, that are made, wholly or in part, from white flour. His diet also was higher in fruits and vegetables than the average and somewhat lower in meats. By avoiding the deficient processed "foods," the diet was

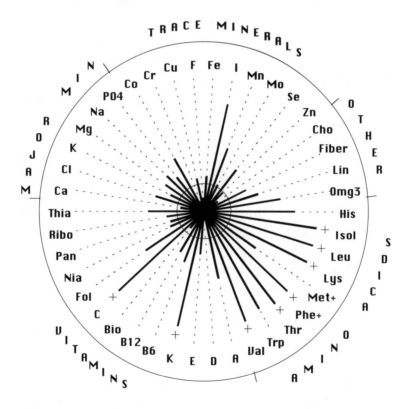

Figure 54. **An individual's diet.** By using available foods and avoiding the use of sugar and white flour products, this individual was able to obtain a diet which is superior to the "average American diet" in all fourteen of the nutrients that are low in the "average."

made far superior to the "average" American diet. In supplying maintenance chemicals, it is superior to the "average" American diet in twenty-six out of forty-two respects. Most importantly, it is superior in all fourteen of the nutrients that are low in the "average" American diet.

What else can each of us do to improve nutrition besides concentrating on good, wholesome foods? Certain kinds of people need to pay particular attention to their nutritional needs. These include pregnant women, small children, teenagers, those with mediocre or poor health, and the elderly. "Average" needs may be irrelevant to their nutrition, and special attention to the details of their nutrition may be most rewarding. One of the measures that can be taken to help ensure adequate nutrition and take care of the special needs of such individuals is the use of nutritional supplements. In Chapter 9 of my *Physicians' Handbook of Nutritional Science*, I have discussed fully a nutritional supplement that will help those with more exacting nutritional needs to obtain an adequate quota of the growth and maintenance chemicals. I suggested some minor improvements in my later book, *The Prevention of Alcoholism Through Nutrition*. The following nutrients are suggested in the amounts indicated (tables 3 and 4).

These are not large amounts, and should be safe and harmless to anyone, while at the same time furnishing a good measure of "insurance." This formula is freely available for public use. One firm that has taken the trouble to provide the supplement at reasonable cost is Bronson Pharmaceuticals, St. Louis, MO 63146. Other companies may sell similar products.

In addition to this "insurance" supplement, it may be desirable in individual cases to use, preferably with the advice of a physician or nutritional expert,

TABLE 3

SUGGESTED VITAMIN FORMULATION FOR NUTRITIONAL INSURANCE

Vitamin A	7,500 units
Vitamin D	400 units
Vitamin E	40 units
Vitamin K (Menedione)	2 mg
Ascorbic acid	250 mg
Thiamin	2 mg
Riboflavin	2 mg
Vitamin B_6	3 mg
Vitamin B_{12}	9 mcg
Niacinamide	20 mg
Pantothenic acid	15 mg
Biotin	0.3 mg
Folic acid	0.4 mg
Choline	250 mg
Inositol	250 mg
P-aminobenzoic acid	30 mg
Rutin	200 mg

TABLE 4

SUGGESTED MINERAL FORMULATION FOR NUTRITIONAL INSURANCE

Calcium	250 mg
Phosphate	750 mg (equivalent to 250 mg phosphorus)
Magnesium	200 mg
Iron	15 mg
Zinc	15 mg
Copper	2 mg
Iodine	0.15 mg
Manganese	5 mg
Molybdenum	0.1 mg
Chromium	1.0 mg
Selenium	0.02 mg
Cobalt	0.1 mg

larger doses of any or all the B vitamins and vitamin C. Some physicians advocate, on occasion, "megadoses" of various B vitamins. These are doses perhaps a hundred or more times the supposed average requirement. In Canada folic acid is available without prescription at much higher levels than is allowed in the U.S. Five milligrams per day should be safe for anyone unless they are threatened with pernicious anemia. A substantial amount of trial and error is involved in the use of larger amounts of supplements. No one who is not an expert should try the use of higher levels of the trace elements.

If you are concerned about heart disease (men are particularly susceptible), the use of nutritional supplements is advised. Certainly they are advised, with moderation, during pregnancy. Unless children are restricted to good, wholesome foods, they should be furnished an insurance supplement. The same is true of the elderly.

If you live in an industrial community and are afraid of cancer induced by industrial chemicals, you will be well advised to use nutritional supplements. It has been convincingly demonstrated that nutritional factors protect against the effects of carcinogens. Good nutrition is also known to protect against other health problems arising because of a polluted environment.

Use of nutritional supplements is certainly advisable as a preventive of mental disease and alcoholism. Large numbers of people who escape mental disease most of their lives suffer from it in the years of their physiological decline with age. It often takes a long period of drinking to produce an alcoholic, and the fact that a person has consumed alcohol with impunity for many years is no assurance that he or she may not become addicted later in life. Observing the rules of good nutrition will prevent anyone from becoming an alcoholic because the rules of good nutrition forbid heavy drinking. The use of nutritional supplements is certainly a potent way of helping to prevent the development of this dread disease. L-glutamine (two to four grams a day) should be included in the nutritional supplement of those seriously threatened with alcoholism. In many cases, this particular amino acid helps greatly to curb the appetite for alcohol. It is quite safe and may have additional benefits.

Some individuals, of course, are capable of consuming food rather carelessly during their adult lives without suffering obvious harm. This makes it more difficult to "sell" the importance of good nutrition to the general public. A person may argue to himself, "If some people get along without much concern for their nutrition, I can afford to be careless." This argument neglects the vital fact of individuality. Incidentally, it has not been demonstrated that anyone can thrive on poor nutrition *starting during his or her developmental years.*

Responses to other environmental factors also differ greatly from person to person. Some children brought up in poverty and in unwholesome atmospheres nevertheless turn out to be highly superior members of society. This is one of the facts of life, but it should not be used as an argument against providing children with good environments.

These facts and those having to do with distinctive nutritional needs should not seem strange to us in the light of material presented in Chapter VI, which demonstrates that anatomically, biochemically, and neurologically we all show remarkable distinctiveness.

We have found it easy to demonstrate in our laboratories that even rats exhibit individuality in their nutritional needs. We fed sixty-four male weanling rats of four different strains a diet consisting wholly of enriched white bread. We knew in advance that rats in general cannot thrive on such a poor diet, but we wished to see how greatly individual rats would differ in their responses to it. One rat grew slowly but continuously and lived for over twenty weeks. At the other extreme, another rat failed to grow appreciably and died within the first week. Every rat responded in its own distinctive way. The life spans of the individual rats were 6, 10, 11, 16, 20, 33, 34, 53, 69, 75, 87, 110, 113, 122, and 144 days. Growth varied similarly; weight gains varied from 2 to 212 grams, in a continuous series of intermediate values.

The rat that gained 212 grams and lived 144 days acquired the name Winston Churchill because we thought he had the kind of constitution that would allow him to be careless about his nutrition. This rat did not really thrive on white bread. His life span of 144 days was considerably less than the normal span of about three years (approximately 1100 days). On a good diet at 144 days, also, he would have been much better developed and would have weighed well over 400 grams. Relatively speaking, however, he performed much better than might have been expected on this poor diet. There are "Winston Churchills" in the general population, but prudent people will not build their lives on the assumption that they belong in this category.

It is a common observation that, because of individuality in nutrition, some people consistently consume a little too much food and tend to become obese. Others tend to eat and assimilate not quite enough and to perpetuate their thinness. For many others, the appetite-regulating mechanisms function almost perfectly, with the result that when they eat as they want to, they are neither too fat nor too lean. This is the ideal situation and would probably be attained by more people *if* the quality of their food were kept at a high level and *if* they exercised adequately. Among wild animals, this internal regulation operates effectively. One does not see deer too fat to jump a fence or squirrels too fat to climb a tree. These animals consume good, wholesome foods exclusively. They usually do not have access to some of the foods that humans, in their wisdom (?), select—those containing such ingredients as extra sugar, starch, white flour, and alcohol.

Generally speaking, people should expect to have some nutritional needs that are far from average. Some adults require very little vitamin A; others require several times the supposed average. Some individuals require about one-fourth the estimated adult need for calcium; others need about five times this much. Amino acid needs can be measured with considerable accuracy and vary, on the average, over about a fourfold range. Individuals may have needs for vitamins D, B_6 and B_{12} that are many times the "estimated adult need." Some of these conditions are referred to in scientific circles as "dependencies." The term applies to a requirement that sticks out like a sore thumb, because it is enormously above average. (The use of the word "dependencies" is unfortunate because we are all dependent on these vitamins.)

The variations cited above are ones that are presently well recognized. There are very likely many others about which we have less definitive information. Nature probably helps us solve some of these problems of individual nutrition more than we realize. We all have some "body wisdom" and we can cultivate it by consuming superior food. Our appetite mechanisms tell us not to eat a pound of butter, drink a glassful of table syrup, or down a tablespoon of salt. If our appetite mechanisms are well nourished and in excellent working order, they probably tell us much more. They tell us, if we but listen, to diversify and not to eat, monotonously, one single food; they probably help us avoid foods that would throw us out of balance; and they help us obtain the individual nutrients we need. The probability that our appetite mechanisms can do this is supported by the fact that rats will, by exercising body wisdom, choose a complete assortment of powdered amino acids mixed together in preference to one from which one of the essential amino acids has been omitted.

Human appetite mechanisms, especially when deranged, can be untrustworthy. An alcoholic's appetite mechanism tells him he must have liquor, and a diabetic's mechanism may tell him he needs sugar. In these cases, body wisdom has become body foolishness. The appetite mechanism of a healthy, well-nourished person probably helps him or her avoid food allergies, which have received considerable attention in recent years. Such conditions, if not guarded against, can cause physical and mental illness.

The idea of individuality in nutrition is not new. The father of medicine, Hippocrates, observed that "different sorts of people have different maladies," and the old-time English clinician, Parry of Bath, held that it is "more important to know what sort of patient has a disease than to know what sort of disease a patient has." Lucretius, the Roman, about two thousand years ago said, "What is one man's meat may be another's poison."

No matter what your age or how good or poor your health, or what your individual nutritional needs, you should receive a tremendous psychological lift from the realization that you are not trapped by your present environment. You are not foredoomed to eke out a humdrum existence. A large part of your environment—your internal environment—can be changed dramatically for the better, and there is no facet of your life that cannot be changed and made happier.

You may be able to improve your nutrition vastly on your own. If you have special problems, however, you may need expert help. There is an excellent prospect that in future years physicians, clinical biochemists, and experts in nutrition can help you greatly.

You are not trapped. You can move ahead in terms of mental and physical health. The doors are open.

In summary, the following nutritional insights, related to food quality and use, can be derived from a consideration of the diagrams of foods and food mixtures presented in this chapter.

1. There exists a marvelous unity in nature. The edible tissues of plants and animals of various kinds all are endowed with the same amino acids, minerals, and vitamins as are present in the metabolic machinery of our body cells. Trace elements such as cobalt, chromium, copper, iron, iodine, manganese, molybdenum, selenium, and zinc are common in many forms of life. Such elements as cesium, beryllium, rubidium, titanium, antimony, germanium, thallium, aluminum, tellurium, and bismuth are available but apparently never utilized. Although one could write the formulas for, and build in the laboratory, hundreds of amino acids and vitamin-like structures, nature does not use these; it sticks to the old stand-bys.

2. The edible portions of plants and animal tissues and other natural foods furnish appropriate assortments of most of the maintenance chemicals. These foods include meats, fish, cereals, vegetables, fruits, nuts, eggs, oysters, and mushrooms. If, for example, we eat oranges "to get vitamin C," or bananas because we like them, or watermelon just for fun, we are contributing good nutrition to the cells and tissues of the body by furnishing suitable amounts

of a host of maintenance chemicals. In contrast, if we consume quantities of items such as sugar or alcohol, our diet is impaired in proportion to the amount of energy received in those forms. Such "foods" fail to furnish any maintenance chemicals.

One should not, however, adopt a worshipful attitude toward all natural foods. Honey is a little better nutritionally than sugar, but only slightly better. Many natural foods, as we have seen, contain traces of toxicants which, in large amounts, may be very harmful. Individually, most natural foods have both strengths and weaknesses.

3. Rarely does one encounter anything approaching a perfect food which furnishes every maintenance chemical in completely adequate amounts. This is evident from our charts. For this reason, as well as others, diversification in one's eating is most desirable. Deficiencies in one food are counterbalanced by others, provided that all foods consumed have in them a reasonable balance between energy content and maintenance chemical content. Energy-yielding "foods" such as sugar cannot contribute to adequate nutrition. They can only cause deterioration in our diet.

4. Some types of food are far more costly than others, when costs are calculated on the basis of the energy content and the daily amount required to sustain life. Lettuce, for example, as can be seen in figure 44, is a very high quality food, but the estimated cost, on the basis of 2,500 calories—a day's total supply of energy—is over $31.00. In contrast, the estimated cost of 2,500 calories in the form of wheat (purchased by the bushel) is about 65¢. Purchased as prepared shredded wheat, it costs about $4.25. (Such cost figures should not be taken too seriously, since they differ from locality to locality and from time to time. Nevertheless, it is clear that, regardless of price

fluctuations, cost figures for different types of foods vary widely.) Although cost is one factor to be considered in choosing foods, it is often subordinate to others. Our discussion should certainly not be construed as suggesting that lettuce should be avoided. People in general would probably be better off if they consumed more of it. In no case, however, should lettuce contribute more than a small percentage of one's food energy.

Those types of foods which are usually consumed in small amounts, insofar as number of calories is concerned, may be relatively expensive when considered on an energy-yielding basis. Their use may be fully justified, however, on quite different grounds.

5. Some foods, because they contain relatively large amounts of water and roughage, cannot be used to supply a large part of one's energy needs. Cabbage, while a food of high quality (see figure 41), belongs in this category. In order to obtain 2,500 calories from cabbage, one would have to consume about twenty-five pounds of it.

6. Some wholesome natural foods should not constitute a large portion of one's calorie intake because they contain small amounts of harmful substances.

7. Every food worthy of the name has in it a reasonable balance between energy content and growth and maintenance chemicals and is useful to many kinds of organisms, not to man alone.

XVI

WHAT WE STILL NEED TO LEARN ABOUT NUTRITION

You have already gained, in this book, very important basic insights into what nutrition is all about. You now know why nutrition is necessary and have at least a rough idea of what the nutritional essentials are. You know that we obtain these nutrients from the tissues of plants and animals and understand how many of these essentials work together as a team to make metabolism possible. You know something of the amounts of each nutrient required and that adjustments in the nutritional environment of cells, tissues, and people is always short of perfection and, therefore, always capable of being improved.

Even among scientists who study nutrition, however, there is much more to be learned. We cannot be sure, for example, that our nutritional alphabet is complete. There may be unrecognized trace minerals and undiscovered or unrecognized vitamins. Also, some of the substances we have listed as essentials may possibly be so only in a limited sense. Uncertainties exist about the degree of need for some of the amino acids. Unquestionably, adults need isoleucine, leucine, lysine, methionine, phenylalanine, threonine, tryptophan, and valine. For children, at least, and possibly for adults, histidine and arginine may some day be added to the list. Editor's note 1998: histidine is added to the list in this edition (see Appendix III). In fact, all the amino acids commonly contained in proteins are of some nutritional benefit, even though some can be dispensed with without seriously impairing bodily functions. The inclusion or

205

exclusion of some of the suggested candidates for vitamin status is a matter of judgment, and such judgments may change even from month to month. If there are still unknown vitamins or other essential nutrients, this constitutes a very serious gap in our knowledge. It means that nutritional experiments up to now are all defective in design because we have worked with an incomplete nutritional chain.

Our knowledge of the functions of some conspicuous nutrients is very incomplete. Most of the B vitamins enter into specific enzymes or enzyme systems, but this is not true of vitamins A, C, or E. In spite of the fact it entered the nutritional picture early enough to be assigned the first letter of the alphabet, the functions of vitamin A, aside from those connected with vision, are poorly understood. A remarkable fact, not adequately investigated, is that vitamin A acid (a substance that cannot function in the eyes as vitamin A can) is able to carry out all the nonvisual functions of vitamin A. What these functions are is largely unknown. They are vital, however; animals cannot reproduce without vitamin A, nor can epithelial tissues maintain their health.

Vitamins C and E appear to be protective substances, preventing unwanted oxidation, but it is unclear why they are so valuable in so many different ways.

One of the enigmas associated with vitamins A, C, and E is why different individuals seem to have enormously different needs for them. If we understood the functions of these vitamins better, we would be far more knowledgeable on this subject.

We also need far more accurate knowledge than we have concerning ranges of needs for nutrients. The Food and Nutrition Board, an arm of the National Research Council, attempts to set up "Recommended Daily Allowances" for an increasing number of nutrients without adequate basic information. To know that a particular amount of a nutrient will satisfy the needs of 90, 95, 98 percent or any other proportion of the population, it would be necessary to have distribution curves showing how the members of a representative population respond to an extensive series of levels. Such distribution curves are rare and inadequate and certainly do not exist for a large number of nutrients. In many cases, the range of variation is unknown, and without this knowledge there can, of course, be no information about the distribution within these ranges.

We are also largely in the dark with respect to the various exchanges of nutrients that take place between the different kinds of cells in our bodies. There are nutrients that are not "alphabet items" for the human body because they can be made in some of the tissues of the body. However, these nutrients may be in the "nutritional alphabets" of certain specific cells which cannot make them. Glutamine is such a nutrient. Because it can be made within the body, it is not one of the essential amino acids. However, tissue culture experiments show that it is an indispensable nutrient for some kinds of human cells. The conclusion seems inevitable: glutamine is produced in excess by some cells for the use of others that require it as an essential nutrient.

Many known substances, and possibly some that are unknown, may be nutrients in the same sense that glutamine is. Among the possibilities are other amino acids (e.g., histidine and arginine) and a number of other known metabolites. Specific substances that quite probably are intercellular nutrients of this sort include inositol, lipoic acid, and coenzyme Q. Even the hormones (which are typically produced in the body) may, in a sense, act as intercellular nutrients.

The reason that knowledge about these nutrients is important is because such substances may become important nutrients in the ordinary sense if the cells in the body normally producing them fail in their performance. In the case of glutamine, if the cells and tissues normally producing it are not up to par, the cells that need it may suffer from malnutrition unless the glutamine is ingested in food. It is entirely possible that nutrients of the glutamine type may prove to be of great importance in practical nutrition.

Another gap in our nutritional knowledge is individual digestive deficiencies. It is commonly assumed, for example, that if individuals receive a good assortment of amino acids in their diets, they will automatically receive a good assortment of amino acids. This is valid, however, only if an individual's digestive system works perfectly. Since there is evidence that different people have distinctive patterns of enzyme efficiencies in their digestive tracts, it is possible that an individual might suffer from a specific amino acid deficiency, not because of a deficiency in the protein consumed but rather because of a deficiency in the digestive enzyme apparatus. How important this source of trouble is we do not know.

Closely related to this are problems of absorption. Absorption is not, as I have mentioned before, an automatic process that can always be guaranteed to work perfectly. Specific enzymes are involved. It is highly probable that individuals suffer from nutritional deficiencies primarily because certain nutrients are defectively absorbed.

Like many other aspects of nutrition related to individuality, we know little, in a practical way, about "body wisdoms" and how they differ from individual to individual. We measure I.Q.s but not B.I.Q.s (body intelligence quotients). Body wisdoms related to nutrition may be of many kinds. We know that body wisdom keeps us from eating a shakerful of salt or from going without salt completely, but how well the mechanism (involving the adrenal glands) works in individuals is not known. It is well known that herbivorous animals, which get quantities of potassium from the vegetation they eat, will travel many miles to find salt licks. Their body wisdom tells them that they must have sodium. (They must excrete relatively large quantities of potassium and cannot do so without losing enough sodium to make them sodium-deficient.) Rats have body wisdoms, some of which have been investigated. If rats are offered, under appropriate conditions, a choice between an incomplete mixture of essential amino acids, and one containing the complete assortment, their body wisdom tells them to choose the latter. Do human beings generally, frequently, seldom, or never have the body wisdom to choose foods that contain a specific amino acid for which they have a high requirement? We do not know. Similar questions about other nutrients also need to be answered.

The most important practical problem confronting us in the nutritional field today is that of learning how to determine the specific nutritional needs of individuals. For those who are hale and hearty, this is hardly a pressing problem, but there are so many in our population for whom robust health is elusive that the demand for such information is, and will be, enormous. Typical individuals, as we have seen, have some needs for nutrients that are likely to be far from average. In addition, there are probably millions of atypical people suffering because of undetermined nutritional deficiencies. Dr. Leon Rosenberg of Yale University has called attention to a number of metabolic disorders, discovered in recent years, in which the afflicted individuals have nutritional demands that certainly are not met by routine consumption of available foods.

The obvious measures open to those who wish to learn to determine individual needs include various types of analysis of blood, urine, saliva, hair, sweat, nails, and biopsy specimens, both before and after "loading" with specific nutrients or related chemicals. Determining individual needs will doubtless turn out to be a formidable task, but not nearly as much so as it would be without automated and computer-based equipment. The whole field of nutrition need not be tackled at one time. Probably development will come piece by piece, and it is quite possible that some nutritional deficiencies are rare enough as not to require routine attention.

Somehow we must learn, without question, how to discover an individual's peculiar needs. Many laboratories are engaged in exploring different facets of this problem. We have mentioned a biochemist, Dr. Mary B. Allen, who has been working on this problem for many years and has brought to light several most striking cases. Unfortunately her work has not been published in detail and, hence, is difficult to evaluate.

XVII

WHO NEEDS TO KNOW

Who needs to know the basic story of nutrition—the story we have told in this book? A backhanded answer is implied when we ask, "Who doesn't need to know?"

Physicians, society's official experts on health, need to know this story because it concerns their fundamental business. They clearly do not need a spurious story; they obviously will not be led, as by the nose, by enthusiasts who cannot know more than a fraction of what physicians know about the workings of the human body. Physicians cannot avoid, and should not be expected to avoid, making up their own minds on the vital aspects of nutrition.

If the story, as I have told it, is in error in any essential respect, I am unable to recognize the errors. Experts of all kinds are invited to scrutinize it carefully for fundamental flaws.

The basic story is set forth in the following seven propositions, which, I believe, cannot be successfully controverted:

1. The health of our bodies is determined largely by the state of the coordinated cells and tissues within them.

2. These cells and tissues can maintain maximum health only when their immediate environment is well adjusted to their needs.

3. Approximately forty chemicals—environmental factors—are essential to the environments of cells and tissues.

4. These environmental factors (mostly of nutritional origin) are capable of being adjusted in so many

ways—numerous deficiencies and imbalances are possible—that the cellular environments commonly encountered in our bodies (like all other environments in the biological world) are never perfectly adjusted. Practically speaking, therefore, nutritional environments are always capable of being improved.

5. The problem of the attainment of maximum health is further complicated by the fact that different sets of cellular metabolic machinery, in different individuals, are by inheritance distinctive. Hence, for optimal health and performance, the cells and tissues of individual persons require distinctive nutritional environments.

6. When one accidentally or intentionally pollutes his internal environment with foreign substances, these interfere with normal nutritional processes. In some cases, at least, improved nutritional environments protect against pollution.

7. Nutrition cannot, therefore, be dismissed by vague references to "balanced diets"; it must become a major theme of scientific exploration.

This story of nutrition is simple enough, in outline, so that it can be understood not only by physicians— the qualified experts—but also by nurses and paramedical personnel and by students long before their studies take them into the fields of public health, medicine, or dentistry. Laymen who never expect to study seriously in these fields will also find the material we have presented understandable and applicable to their own lives.

Food producers, processors, manufacturers, and dealers constitute a group with a special need to know the story of nutrition, as we have told it. Currently, the primary interest of those who deal in food is its appearance, taste, and keeping quality. This is supported by slick advertising which exploits nutritional illiteracy. The objective of performing a public service by furnishing food of high quality for children and adults is a minor consideration and is most often pursued, if at all, largely in ignorance.

Several years ago in our laboratories we made comparative tests on the nutritional quality of commercial "enriched" white bread and the same bread to which was added small, inexpensive amounts of other nutrients conspicuously lacking in this important staple food. The results were startling; on the average, young experimental animals grew and developed seven times as fast on the supplemented bread as on the commercial product.

These experiments suggest that the dominant interest in the baking industry is to produce bread that is attractive in taste and texture, regardless of its basic nutritional value. While some bakers are interested in producing breads of higher nutritional quality, the giants in the industry have been very slow to move in that direction. More recently, however, the Food and Nutrition Board has advocated doing a far better job of "enriching" white flour and bread.

Many factors underlie the operations of the food industry that do not appear on the surface. For example, the production of a highly nutritious bread with good keeping qualities and high acceptability to the public taste is not a simple matter, by any means. It is a job for nutritional and technical experts. In other industries—telephone, electronics, computers, glass, business machines, paint, paper, and others— many of the best-qualified experts are to be found within the industries themselves. The lack of competent nutritional experts in the food industry, however, is conspicuous.

Inexpertness in the food industry is exemplified by the recent production and sale of an egg substitute which, when tested for its biological food value, seemed sorely deficient. Professor Kummerow of the University of Illinois has given me permission to present a picture (figure 55) of two rats of the same age fed in his laboratories. The one on the left and its lactating mother were fed hen-laid eggs; the one on the right and its lactating mother received the commercial egg substitute. The comparison speaks for itself. If it is desirable to produce an egg substitute containing no cholesterol (the advantage of this, in my opinion, is *extremely* dubious), then experts should certainly be able to come up with something vastly better than this product. We fear, however, that the producers were thinking mostly of taste, texture, and appearance, and gave little thought to food quality. Imagine

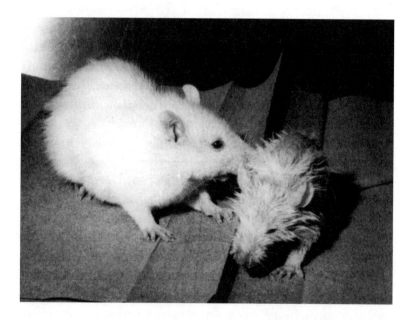

Figure 55. Two rats of the same age. The one on the left and its lactating mother were fed egg, the one on the right and its lactating mother, a commercial egg substitute. The disheveled condition of the rat on the right may be owing in part to the fact that the egg substitute stuck in its hair. However, it is well known that animals fed poorly balanced diets often fail to groom themselves.

feeding a young child this egg substitute on the supposition that it would be equivalent to real eggs!

Parents need to know the story of nutrition because their children's future may hinge on the quality of the food they receive. It is absolutely impossible for a child to develop to its full potential unless the brain and all the other tissues receive the right kind of nourishment. The mere fact that a child continues to live without serious overt disease does not prove that he or she is getting acceptable nutrition. Our animal friends, Peewee and Puny, continued to live, even though the nutrition furnished them was of very low quality.

Teachers and all those entrusted with the care and development of children also need to know the story of nutrition so that they can use all the available resources to achieve their objectives. Those who are concerned with learning difficulties need to know about nutrition because it may offer a key to real help. Psychologists, counselors, ministers, and others who advise people in emergencies need to know the story of nutrition because this facet of the environment may be crucially important in the resolution of difficulties.

Youngsters, themselves, need to know the story of nutrition. This is why we have included high school students in our audience and have prepared a book that can be read by them. In a few short years, the high school students of today will be tomorrow's doctors, dentists, teachers, counselors, ministers, and advisors. They need to be well nourished if they are to be the kind of leaders we need.

Athletes, faddists, senior citizens, and all others who eat need to know the basic facts about nutrition. In addition, there are two special groups that may profit in unique ways from a good understanding of the possibilities that lie ahead in nutritional science.

In one such group are the manufacturers and

users of automated laboratory equipment and accessories. I predict that in the years ahead an industry employing many thousands and rendering services for which people will gladly pay many billions, will be centered around the need of individuals to know, with some assurance, what their peculiar nutritional needs are. I receive large numbers of inquiries emphatically suggesting that there is already a substantial demand. As the story of nutrition becomes better known, that demand will increase enormously. People in affluent circumstances will be served first, and their willingness to pay for help will pave the way for broader application. There is almost no limit to the eventual size of this industry.

Another special group needing desperately to know the story of nutrition and its application to individuals include those concerned with problems of alcoholism and drug addiction. Although it is true that many people are capable of becoming drug addicts or alcoholics, the basic idea that it is *man* who becomes addicted is most misleading. Vulnerabilities to these afflictions vary enormously from person to person. Certain individuals with unusual metabolic characteristics and nutritional needs are in peculiar danger, and progress in solving these problems has been seriously hampered because so little attention has been paid to individual needs. I am convinced that a great opportunity lies waiting for those in this field who are prepared to consider very seriously the impact that nutrition may have. When alcoholics, as a group, are familiar with the story of nutrition, they will be among those most anxious to learn what their own peculiar individual nutritional needs are.

Drug addiction and individual nutrition have never been seriously considered together. It is entirely possible that nutritional factors play a highly significant role in drug addiction and that improved individual nutrition can play a leading part in the rehabilitation of drug addicts.

I am still interested in the partnership proposed in Chapter II. I hope my readers will now be enthusiastic about spreading the word about good nutrition and all of its potentialities. I hope they will keep informed themselves, inform others, and do everything else in their power to see that the long neglected truths in this field are at last given a full-scale opportunity to benefit humanity.

Appendix I

A Few Suggestions About Further Study

The material in this Appendix is primarily for the use of younger readers—those who have not yet finished their formal education but may be seriously attracted to the field of nutrition. These young readers may be the leaders of tomorrow; they may well be the ones who will take most seriously the partnership I suggested in Chapter II.

Our discussions in this book have been largely nontechnical. If one is to become proficient in nutrition, however, it will be necessary to become technical and to acquire a working grasp of how, in detail, metabolism works and how the nutrients mesh together in the machinery that makes cellular life possible.

The first essential for those who seek proficiency in nutritional science is a good understanding of the fundamentals of chemistry. This is a formidable but exciting task. Study in school, reading outside of school, and individual concentration and thought are important ways of making progress.

To emphasize the importance of chemistry as a sound foundation on which to build a knowledge of nutrition, I have included Appendix II with structural formulas and symbols for all the known maintenance chemicals and a number of other chemical structures commonly found in living cells. Very little if any benefit will be derived from rote memorization of the formulas as presented. In order to be proficient in nutrition, one needs to know their meaning, how every meaningful detail has been ascertained, and what kinds of chemical transformations are made possible as the result of these molecules having the structures they have been found experimentally to have. This calls for a good grounding in organic chemistry.

Biology is another field with which one must get a working knowledge if one is to delve deeply into nutritional science. This subject is easier to study outside of school than is chemistry. Biology does not involve concentration on learning the names of all kinds of organisms, or the names of all sorts of anatomical details. It is far more important to gain insight, at the cellular and molecular level, into how diverse organisms carry on their operations such as digestion, assimilation, circulation, metabolism, and excretion.

Biology has many facets. Psychology is fundamentally a branch of biology and is one of the fields in which nutritional experts should have some competence. Statistics is another vitally important area. I suggest that you concentrate on those aspects of biology which mean something to *you* and capture your interest. Because of the diversity of human minds, you will probably find the presentations of some authors more appealing than others. It is important, I believe, for you to take time for "thinking parties," just to entertain and pamper some of your own thoughts and deliberations.

The following books on biology, written for college-level students, are among the better ones available [updated by D. R. Davis]:

Mader, Sylvia S., *Biology* (6th ed.). W. C. Brown/McGraw-Hill, Dubuque, Iowa, 1997.

Raven, Peter H. and Johnson, George B., *Biology* (4th ed.). W. C. Brown, Dubuque, Iowa, 1996.

Campbell, Neil A., *Biology* (4th ed.). Benjamin/Cummings Pub. Co., Menlo Park, California, 1996.

If you like the presentation given in the main body of this book, you may want to read others of my books that have some bearing on nutrition: *Nutrition in a Nutshell* (Doubleday Dolphin Books, a paperback written in 1962); *Biochemical Individuality* (published originally by John Wiley & Sons in 1956, now available in paperback from Keats Publishing, New Canaan, Connecticut, 1998 edition); *Alcoholism: The Nutritional Approach* (University of Texas Press, 1959); *You are Extraordinary* (Random House, 1967, Pyramid paperback edition, Pyramid Press, 1971); *Nutrition Against Disease* (Pitman, 1971; Keats Publishing, New Canaan, Connecticut, 1998 printing planned); *Physicians' Handbook of Nutritional Science* (C. C. Thomas, 1975); and *The Prevention of Alcoholism Through Nutrition* (Bantam Books, 1981).

The following are three widely used books on biochemistry which may be consulted and studied:

Horton, H. Robert, *Principles of Biochemistry* (2nd ed.). Prentice Hall, New Jersey, 1996.

Zubay, Geoffrey L., *Principles of Biochemistry*. W. C. Brown, Dubuque, Iowa, 1995.

Smith, Emil L., Hill, Robert L., Lehman, I. Robert, Lefkowitz, Robert J., Handler, Philip, and White, Abraham, *Principles of Biochemistry* (7th ed.). McGraw-Hill, New York, 1983.

One of the recent books on biochemistry–*Textbook of Biochemistry*, edited by Thomas M. Devlin (Wiley-Liss, New York, 1992)–makes at least one move to emphasize the importance of nutrition. Two chapters are on this subject.

These books on biochemistry can be understood only superficially unless you have a good foundation in chemistry, including organic chemistry. The importance of reading *critically* whatever you read in science can scarcely be overemphasized. This means understanding what you read, thinking as you go along, and incorporating what you read into forming your own opinions and judgments. Merely reading passively without putting yourself into what you read is of little benefit.

Old-line books on nutrition cannot be recommended by me as being very helpful. This is because they fail to present the newer and highly illuminating insights. However, if you can find any books on nutrition that do justice to the important principles stressed throughout this book, I recommend that you study them thoroughly.

Appendix II

Structural formulas and symbols for human nutritional alphabet items cited in Appendix I
(Listed in alphabetical groups as on page 28)

Amino Acids

$$HC \underset{HN-CH}{\overset{N}{=}} C-CH_2-CH \begin{array}{c} C-OH \\ || \\ O \end{array} \quad NH_2$$

Histidine (α-amino-β-imidazolepropionic acid or β-imidazolealanine)

$$CH_3-CH_2-\underset{}{\overset{CH_3}{\underset{|}{CH}}}-\underset{NH_2}{\overset{}{\underset{|}{CH}}}-C-OH \quad (O)$$

Isoleucine
(α-amino-β-methylvaleric acid)

$$CH_3-\overset{CH_3}{\underset{|}{CH}}-CH_2-\overset{NH_2}{\underset{|}{CH}}-\overset{O}{\overset{||}{C}}-OH$$

Leucine
(α-aminoisocaproic acid)

$$H_2N-CH_2-CH_2-CH_2-CH_2-\overset{NH_2}{\underset{|}{CH}}-\overset{O}{\overset{||}{C}}-OH$$

Lysine
(α,ε-diaminocaproic acid)

$$CH_3-S-CH_2-CH_2-\overset{\overset{\displaystyle NH_2}{|}}{CH}-\overset{\overset{\displaystyle O}{||}}{C}-OH$$

Methionine
(α-amino-γ-methylthio-n-butyric acid))

$$\text{(ring)}\quad C-CH_2-\overset{\overset{\displaystyle NH_2}{|}}{CH}-\overset{\overset{\displaystyle O}{||}}{C}-OH$$

Phenylalanine
(α-amino-β-phenylpropionic acid or
β-phenylalanine)

$$CH_3-\overset{\overset{\displaystyle OH}{|}}{CH}-\overset{\overset{\displaystyle NH_2}{|}}{CH}-\overset{\overset{\displaystyle O}{||}}{C}-OH$$

Threonine
(α-amino-β-hydroxy-n-butyric acid)

$$\text{(ring)}\quad C-CH_2-\overset{\overset{\displaystyle NH_2}{|}}{CH}-\overset{\overset{\displaystyle O}{||}}{C}-OH$$

Tryptophan
(α-amino-β-indolepropionic acid or β-indolealanine)

$$CH_3-\overset{\overset{\displaystyle CH_3}{|}}{CH}-\overset{\overset{\displaystyle NH_2}{|}}{CH}-\overset{\overset{\displaystyle O}{||}}{C}-OH$$

Valine
(α-aminoisovaleric acid)

224

Major Minerals

Ca^{++}	Cl^-	K^+
Calcium Ion	Chloride Ion	Potassium Ion
Mg^{++}	Na^+	PO_4^{---}
Magnesium Ion	Sodium Ion	Phosphate Ion

Trace Minerals

Co	Cr	Cu	F
Cobalt	Chromium	Copper	Fluorine
Fe	I	Mn	Mo
Iron	Iodine	Manganese	Molybdenum
	Se	Zn	
	Selenium	Zinc	

Since the exact ionic forms for these trace minerals are not known in all cases, we have indicated them all as the elements themselves.

Vitamins

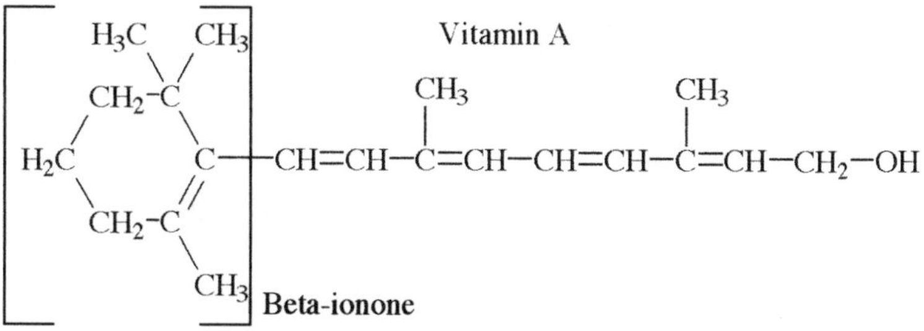

Vitamin A

Beta-ionone

Vitamin A$_1$

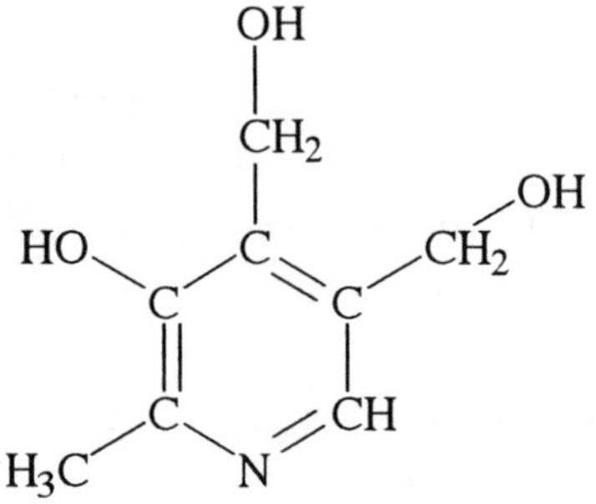

Pyridoxine

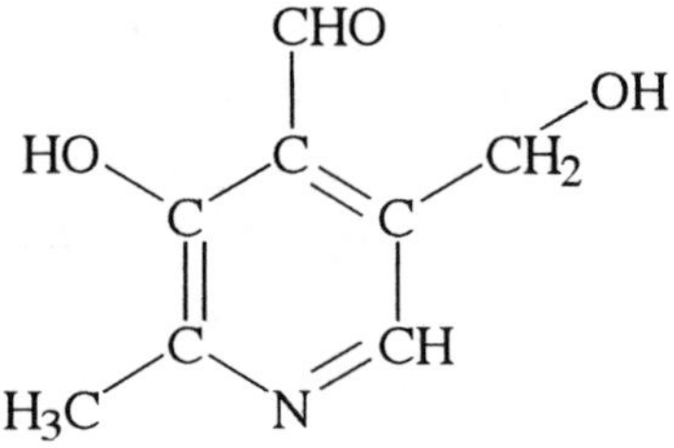

Pyridoxal

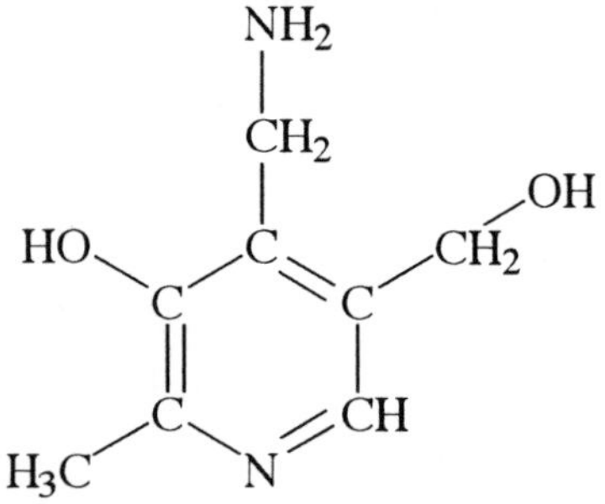

Pyridoxamine

Vitamin B$_6$ (three forms)

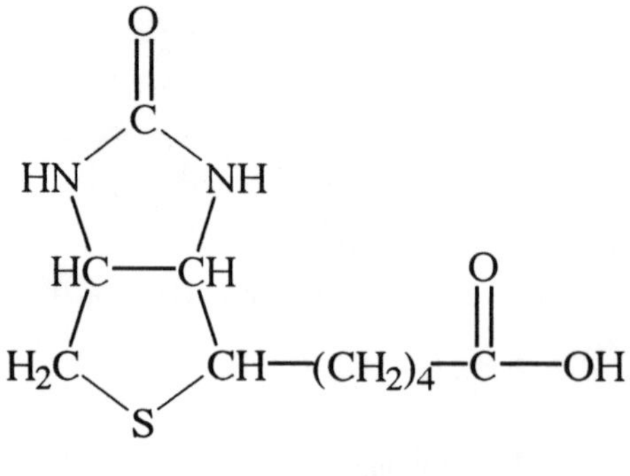

Biotin

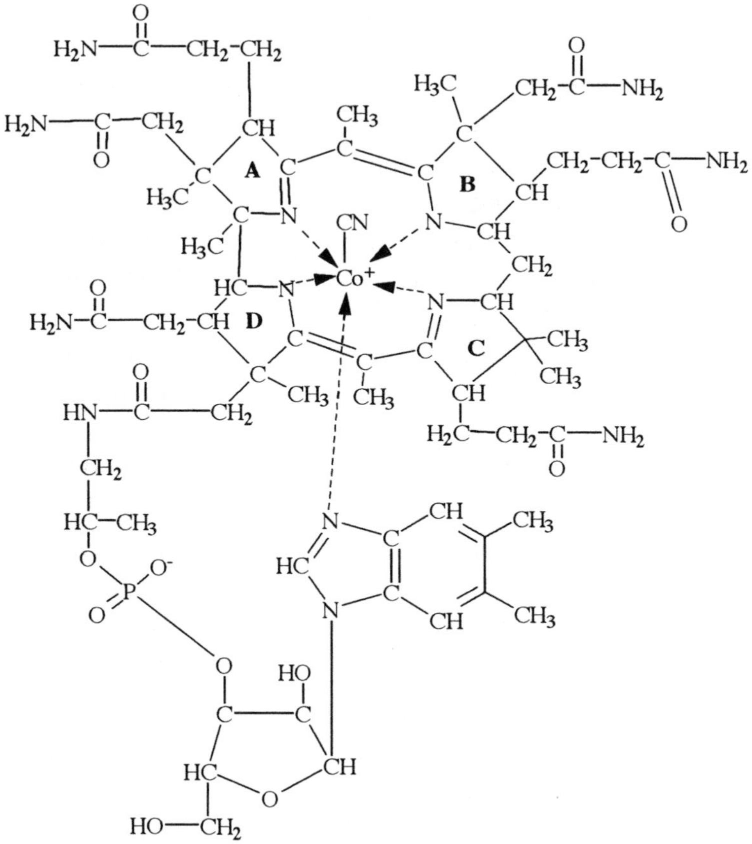

Vitamin B$_{12}$

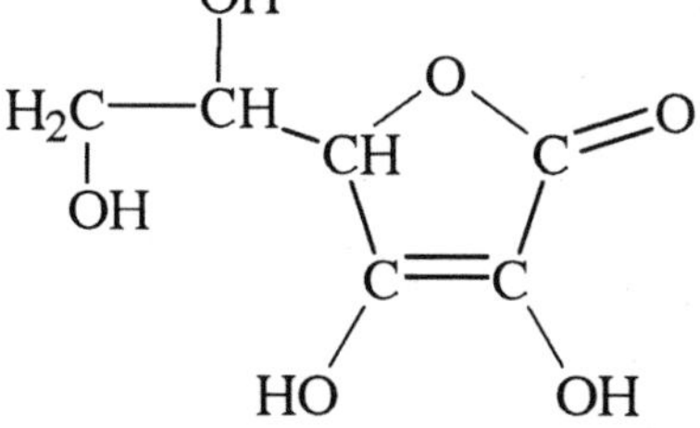

Vitamin C
Ascorbic Acid

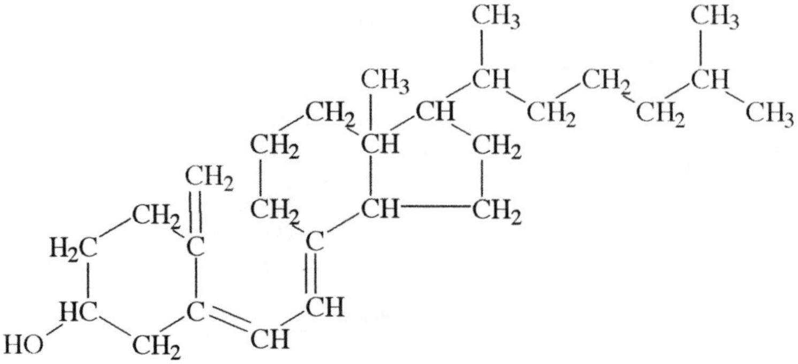

Vitamin D$_3$

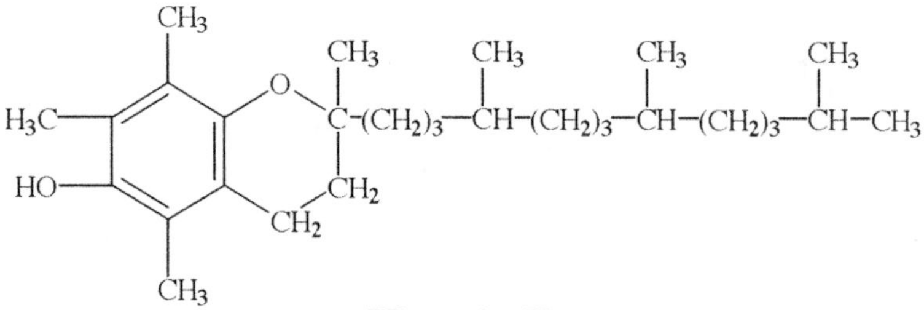

Vitamin E
α-Tocopherol

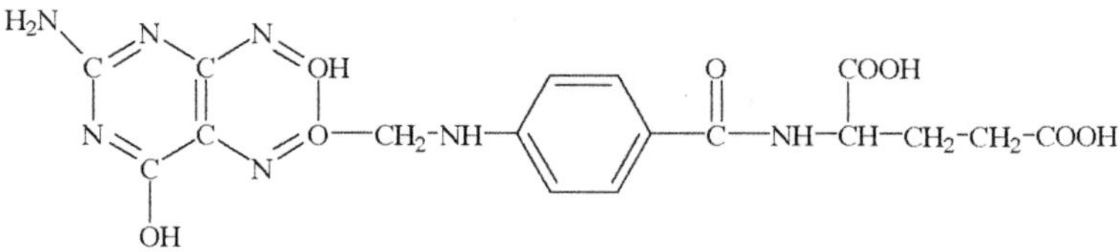

Folic Acid

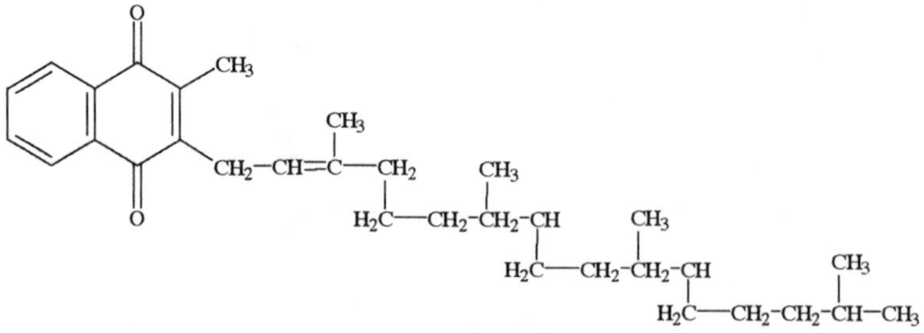

Vitamin K$_1$

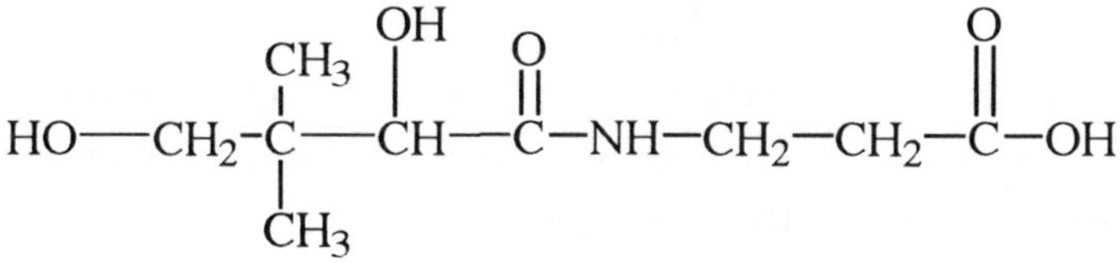

Pantothenic acid (pantoyl-β-alanine)

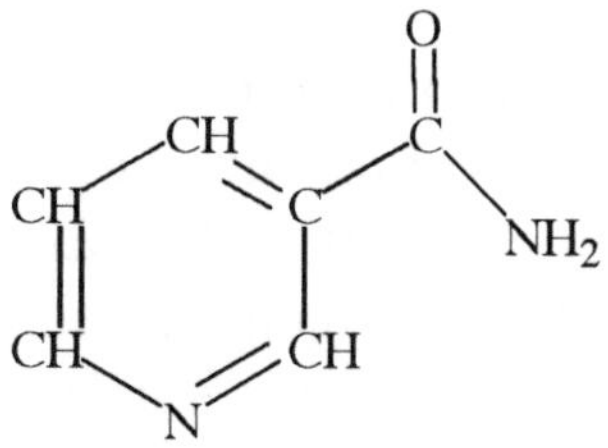

Niacinamide
Nicotinamide

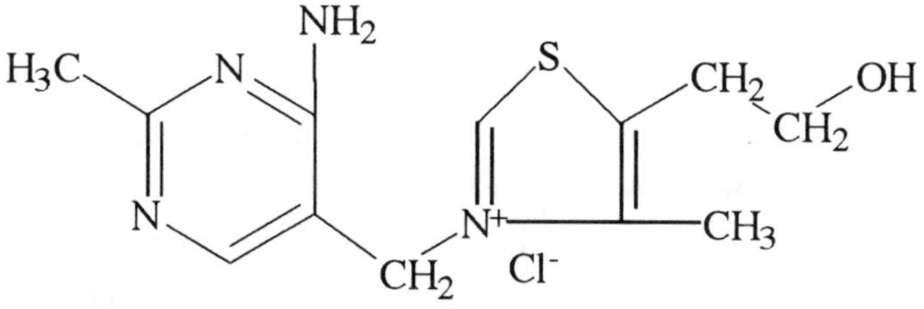

Vitamin B$_1$
Thiamin hydrochloride

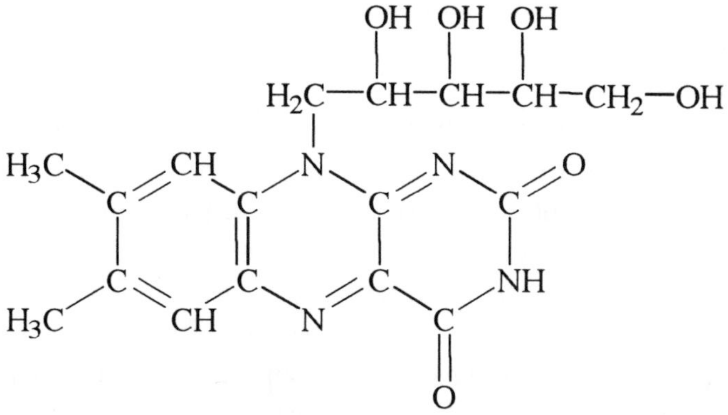

Riboflavin

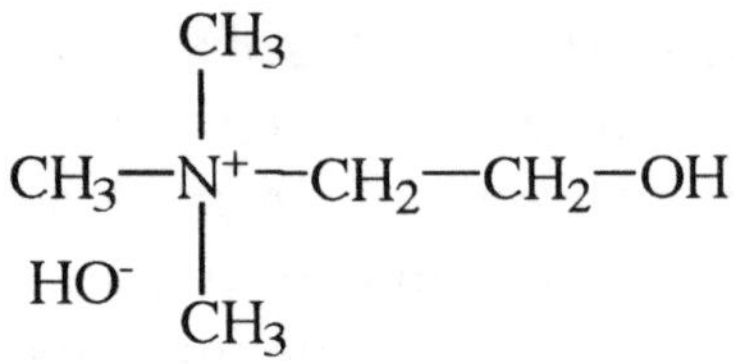

$$CH_3-\overset{\overset{\displaystyle CH_3}{|}}{\underset{\underset{\displaystyle CH_3}{|}}{N^+}}-CH_2-CH_2-OH$$

HO⁻

Choline

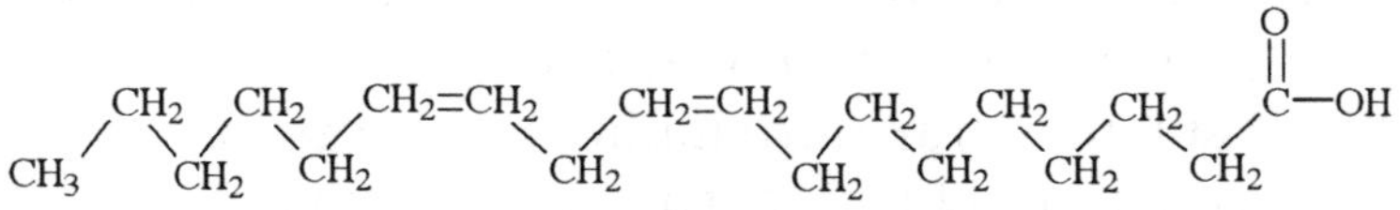

$$CH_3 \diagup CH_2 \diagup CH_2 \diagup CH_2{=}CH_2 \diagup CH_2{=}CH_2 \diagup CH_2 \diagup CH_2 \diagup CH_2 \diagup \overset{\overset{\displaystyle O}{\|}}{C}-OH$$

Linoleic acid

$$CH_3 \diagdown CH{=}CH \diagup CH{=}CH \diagup CH{=}CH \diagup CH_2 \diagup CH_2 \diagup CH_2 \diagup \overset{\overset{\displaystyle O}{\|}}{C}-OH$$

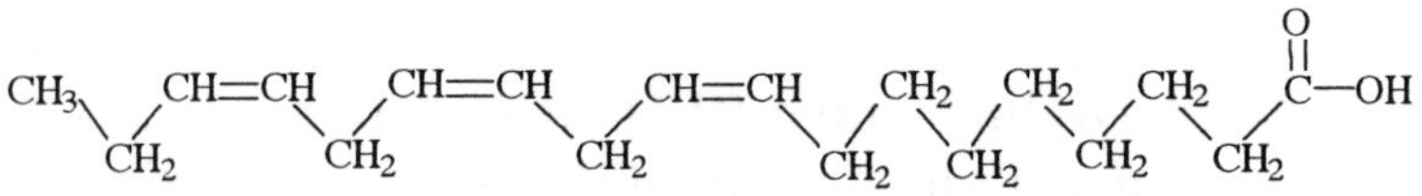

Alpha Linolenic acid

Other cellular constituents ordinarily produced internally: they do not have to be furnished to human beings by the nutritional environment.

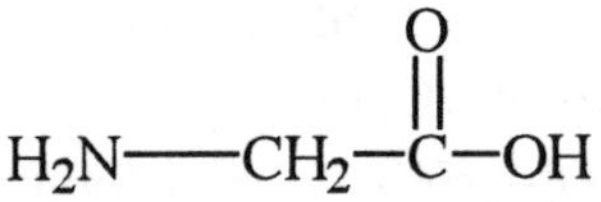

$$H_2N\text{——}CH_2-\overset{\overset{\displaystyle O}{\|}}{C}-OH$$

Glycine (aminoacetic acid)

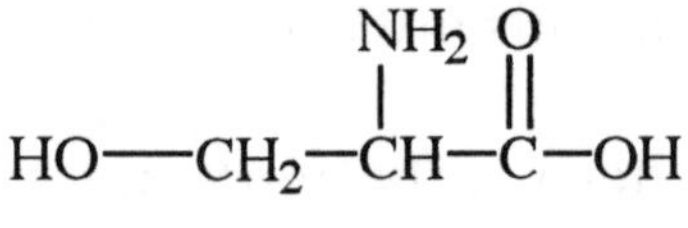

$$HO-CH_2-\overset{\overset{\displaystyle NH_2}{|}}{CH}-\overset{\overset{\displaystyle O}{\|}}{C}-OH$$

Serine
(α-amino-β-hydroxypropionic acid, β-hydroxyalanine)

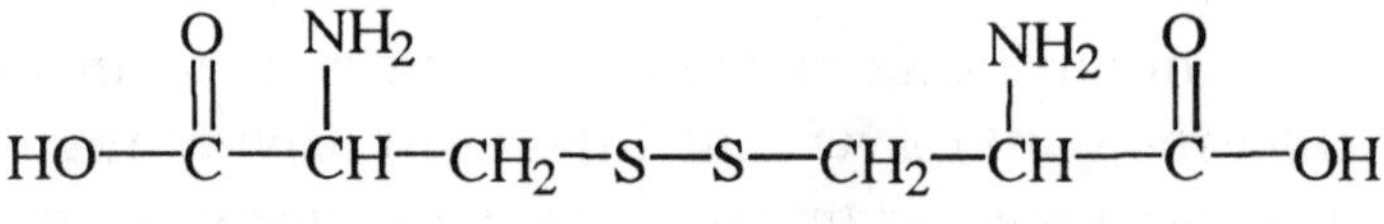

$$HO-\overset{\overset{\displaystyle O}{\|}}{C}-\overset{\overset{\displaystyle NH_2}{|}}{CH}-CH_2-S-S-CH_2-\overset{\overset{\displaystyle NH_2}{|}}{CH}-\overset{\overset{\displaystyle O}{\|}}{C}-OH$$

Cystine (di-[α-amino-β-thiopropionic acid])

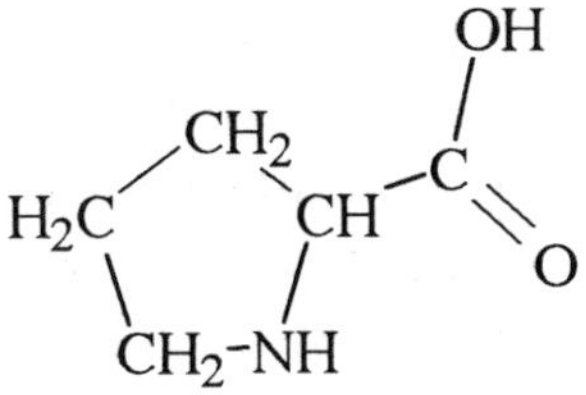

$$H_2C \underset{CH_2-NH}{\overset{CH_2}{\diagdown}} CH-C\overset{OH}{\underset{O}{\diagup}}$$

Proline
(pyrrolidine-2-carboxylic acid)

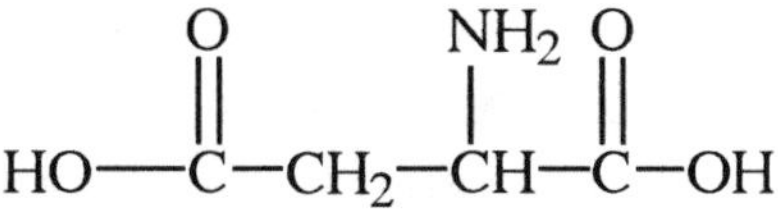

$$HO-\overset{O}{\overset{\|}{C}}-CH_2-\overset{NH_2}{\overset{|}{CH}}-\overset{O}{\overset{\|}{C}}-OH$$

Aspartic acid
(aminosuccinic acid)

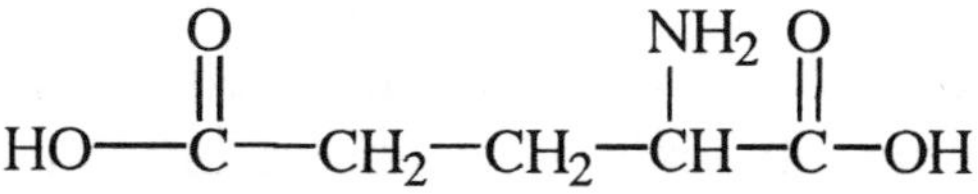

$$HO-\overset{O}{\overset{\|}{C}}-CH_2-CH_2-\overset{NH_2}{\overset{|}{CH}}-\overset{O}{\overset{\|}{C}}-OH$$

Glutamic acid (α-aminoglutaric acid)

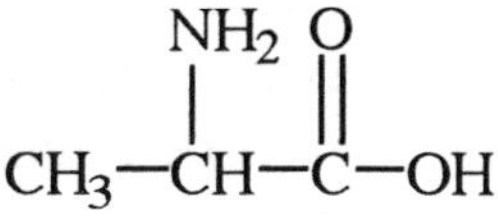

$$CH_3-\overset{NH_2}{\overset{|}{CH}}-\overset{O}{\overset{\|}{C}}-OH$$

Alanine (α-aminoproprionic acid)

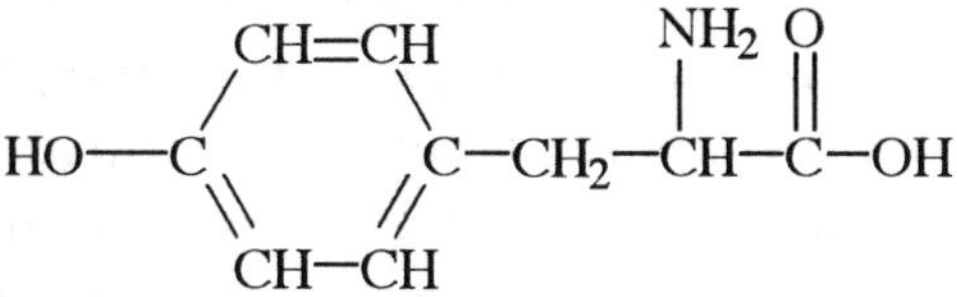

$$HO-\overset{CH=CH}{\underset{CH-CH}{\diagup\diagdown}} C-CH_2-\overset{NH_2}{\overset{|}{CH}}-\overset{O}{\overset{\|}{C}}-OH$$

Tyrosine (α-amino-β-[p-hydroxyphenyl]
propionic phenylalanine)

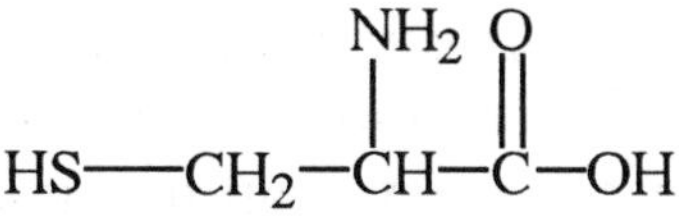

$$HS-CH_2-\overset{NH_2}{\overset{|}{CH}}-\overset{O}{\overset{\|}{C}}-OH$$

Cysteine
(α-amino-β-
mercaptopropionic acid)

$$\underset{\substack{\text{HO} \quad \quad \quad \text{CH} \\ | \quad \quad \quad | \\ \text{CH}_2\text{-NH}}}{\overset{\substack{\text{OH} \\ | \\ \text{CH}_2 \quad \quad \text{C} \\ \diagup \quad \diagdown \quad \diagup \diagdown \\ \text{CH} \quad \quad \text{CH} \quad \text{O}}}{}}$$

Hydroxyproline
(4-hydroxypyrrolidine-2-carboxylic acid,
or oxyproline)

$$\text{H}_2\text{N}\!-\!\!\overset{\overset{\text{O}}{\|}}{\text{C}}\!-\!\text{CH}_2\!-\!\overset{\overset{\text{NH}_2}{|}}{\text{CH}}\!-\!\overset{\overset{\text{O}}{\|}}{\text{C}}\!-\!\text{OH}$$

Asparagine, the β-amide of aspartic acid

$$\text{H}_2\text{N}\!-\!\!\overset{\overset{\text{O}}{\|}}{\text{C}}\!-\!\text{CH}_2\!-\!\text{CH}_2\!-\!\overset{\overset{\text{NH}_2}{|}}{\text{CH}}\!-\!\overset{\overset{\text{O}}{\|}}{\text{C}}\!-\!\text{OH}$$

Glutamine, the γ-amide of glutamic acid

$$\text{H}_2\text{N}\!-\!\text{CH}_2\!-\!\overset{\overset{\text{OH}}{|}}{\text{CH}}\!-\!\text{CH}_2\!-\!\text{CH}_2\!-\!\overset{\overset{\text{NH}_2}{|}}{\text{CH}}\!-\!\overset{\overset{\text{O}}{\|}}{\text{C}}\!-\!\text{OH}$$

Hydroxylysine (α,ε-diamino-δ-hydroxycaproic acid)

$$\text{H}_2\text{N}\!-\!\!\overset{\overset{\text{NH}}{\|}}{\text{C}}\!-\!\text{NH}\!-\!\text{CH}_2\!-\!\text{CH}_2\!-\!\text{CH}_2\!-\!\overset{\overset{\text{NH}_2}{|}}{\text{CH}}\!-\!\overset{\overset{\text{O}}{\|}}{\text{C}}\!-\!\text{OH}$$

Arginine (α-amino-δ-guanidovaleric acid)

$$\underset{\substack{\text{O}=\text{C} \quad \quad \text{CH} \\ \diagdown \quad \diagup \\ \text{NH}}}{\overset{\substack{\text{NH}_2 \\ | \\ \text{C} \\ \diagup \diagdown \\ \text{N} \quad \quad \text{CH} \\ \| \quad \quad \|}}{}}$$

Cytosine (2-Oxy-4-aminopyrimidine)

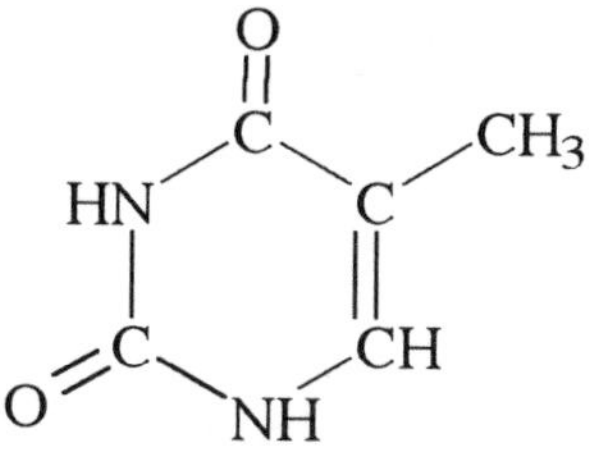

Thymine
(5-Methyl-2,4-dioxypyrimidine)

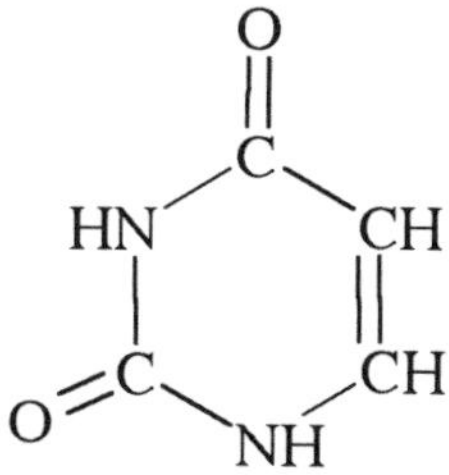

Uracil (2,4-Dioxypyrimidine)

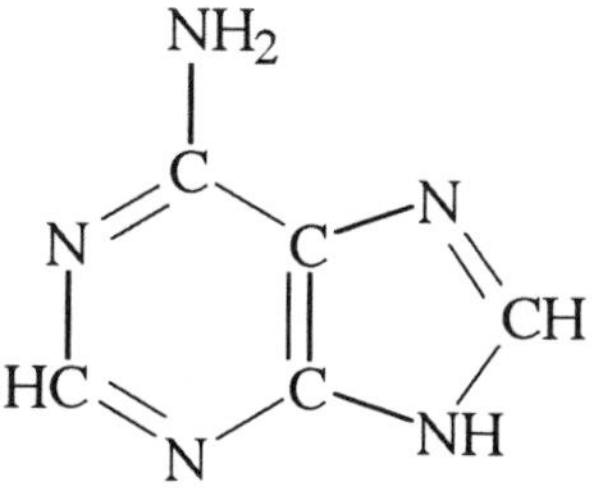

Adenine (6-Aminopurine) 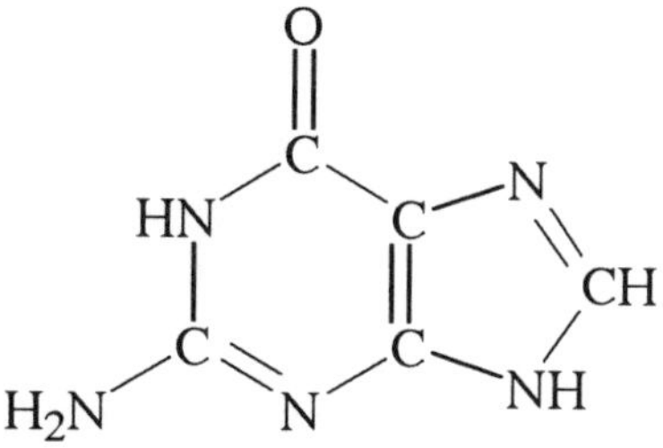 *Guanine* (2-Amino-6-oxypurine)

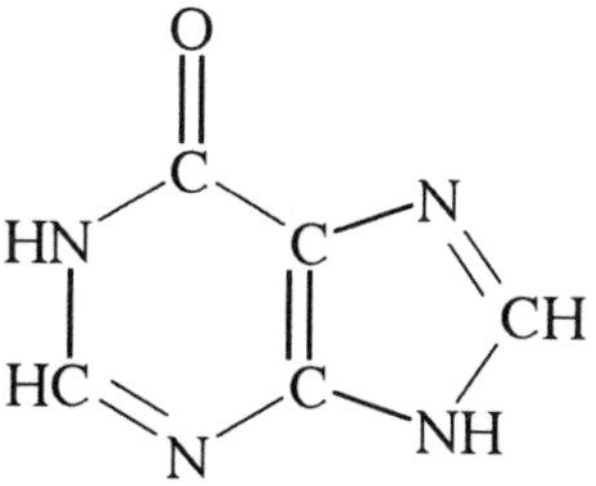

Hypoxanthine
(6-Oxypurine)

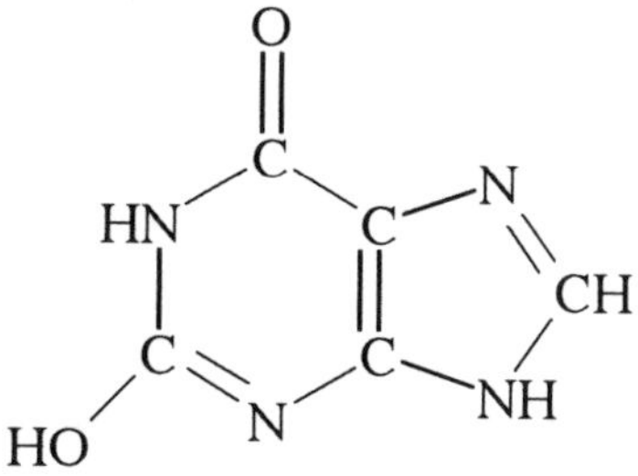

Xanthine
(2,6-Dioxypurine)

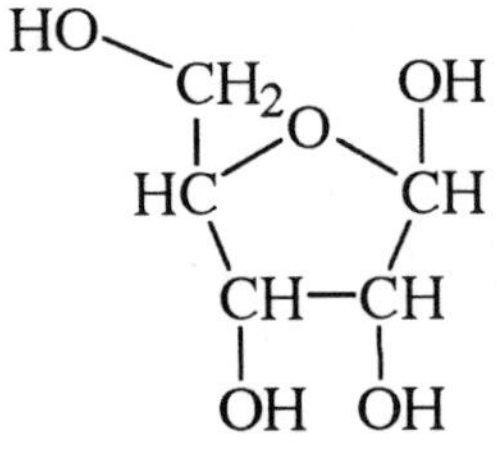

D-Ribose
(α-D-ribofuranose)

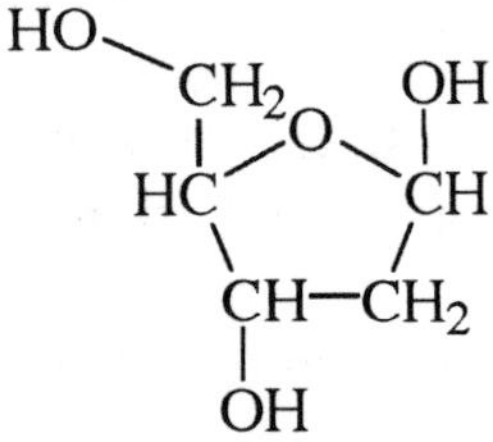

D-2-Deoxyribose
(α-D-2-deoxyribofuranose)

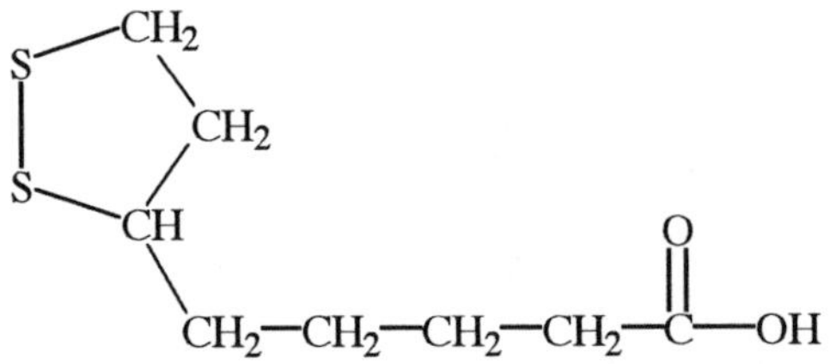

α-*Lipoic acid* (6,8-dithio-n-octanoic acid)

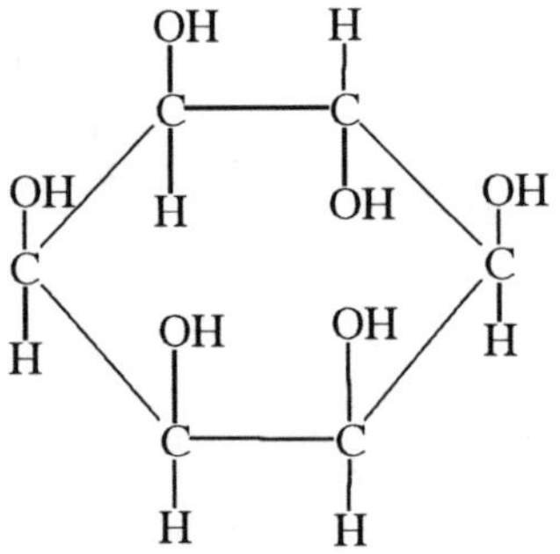

Inositol

Appendix III
Notes for Table 1,
List of Growth and Maintenance
Chemicals

by Donald R. Davis, Ph.D.

Three items in Table 1 are new to the 1998 edition: omega-3 fatty acids, histidine, and dietary fiber. Their essential status was not established when the book first appeared in 1977, or in the case of dietary fiber, too little was known about the amounts in foods and the amounts needed.

The estimated adult daily requirements for most items in Table 1 have been reduced from the 1977 and 1987 editions, based primarily on new information about the amounts in wholesome diets. The largest change is for chromium which we now know requires special precautions to prevent laboratory contamination of food samples from stainless steel and other sources. Amounts in uncontaminated foods average about 10 times less than was previously reported, so the recommended amount in Table 1 is 10 fold less than before.

The other largest changes are for selenium (now 8 fold less), vitamin K (7 fold less), cobalt (5 fold less) and biotin (4 fold less). All of these items are still much less studied than most others in the table.

Two changes in this edition reflect changes in the current (1989) U. S. Recommended Dietary Allowances (RDAs), and are less likely than the other changes to have been endorsed by Williams. These are for vitamin E (now 3 fold less) and folic acid (2 fold less). Much new evidence since 1989 supports increasing the RDAs for vitamin E, folic acid, and vitamin C.

INDEX

Free Software Offer

(Free By Internet)

If you like the 40 nutrient diagrams in this book, you will love the enhanced versions for Windows 95. Here's some of what you can do:

- Display color diagrams on your computer
- Change scales to view minor and major nutrients
- Compare two foods side-by-side
- See pie charts with types of calories and types of fat
- Print large diagrams in color or black & white
- Make overhead slides
- Show nutrient amounts in any serving size
- Transfer diagrams to other software

How to get your free software (Windows 95) By Internet:
> http://www.brightspot.org/nutri.html

Also available by mail (3.5-inch diskette) for $3.95 shipping and handling charge. Send check to:
> NutriCircles Software Offer
> The Bright Spot for Health
> 3100 N. Hillside Ave.
> Wichita, Kansas 67219

You will receive a special edition of NutriCircles® software created for readers of this book. A full version with over 2000 foods is also available by Internet or mail order (1-800-447-7276). It contains many other features you can use to improve your nutrition. These include analysis of meals and recipes, Nutritional Wholeness™ and searching for foods high or low in over 60 nutrients.

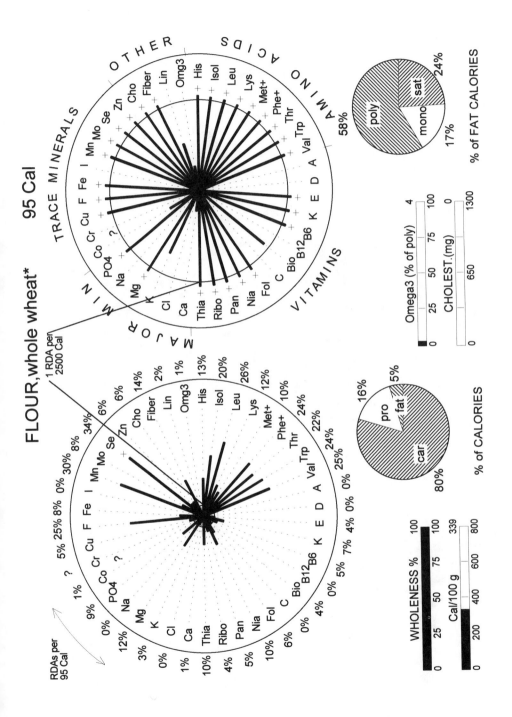

FLOUR, whole wheat*   95 Cal

247

ABOUT THE CENTER

Bio-Communications Press, a service of **The Center for the Improvement of Human Functioning International**, published its first book in 1987. Since that time a variety of books concerning health and nutrition have been published.

The Center, also known as the **Bright Spot for Health**, is located in the heart of the USA in Wichita, Kansas. The campus is situated on 92 acres and contains 8 geodesic 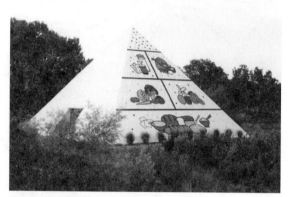 domes and the largest food guide pyramid in the world. The Center began in 1975 as a small nutritional, research/clinical laboratory with a staff of three. Today, The Center is a complex medical, research, and educational organization with several major divisions.

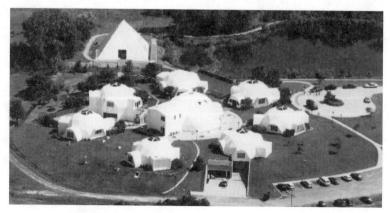

To date, thousands of people from all 50 states, the district of Columbia, and 29 foreign countries have come to the **Olive W. Garvey Center for Healing Arts**. They have come to benefit from our in-depth evaluation and treatment recommendations after not responding to standard medical care. As a driving force for a new emphasis in medicine, The Center is growing in its service and capability for discovering underlying causes of disease. More patients are demanding our type of care based upon nutritional medicine and each individual's unique biochemistry, principles discovered by Dr. Roger Williams. Our medical doctors, therapists, and nurses, with years of experience in diverse specialities, work together as a treatment team to provide coordinated care—the cornerstone of The Center's effectiveness.

The **Bio-Center Laboratory** provides diagnostic services for physicians and hospitals throughout the country to help reveal biochemical impairments and monitor their correction. Advanced instrumentation, including computerized atomic absorption and plasma spectrometry, gas chromatography, high pressure liquid chromatography, spectrophotometry, spectro-fluorometry and gamma counter analyzers, provides the laboratory with a resource for complex test procedures. All assays are performed by highly-skilled technologists and technicians using precision quality control techniques to ensure their accuracy. The Bio-Center Laboratory has received continuous certification from state and federal agencies since 1976.

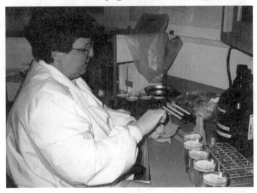

The **Mabee Library** is a respected medical research library utilized by patients, staff, researchers, students, and the public. Though not a lending library, over 4,000 books, 2,500 au-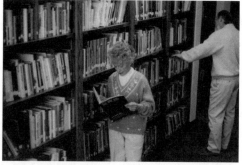dio tapes, 750 videos, and 150 journals and newsletters are available for use. The library is an integral part of the **Bio-Medical Synergistics Education Institute**. This division provides learning opportuni-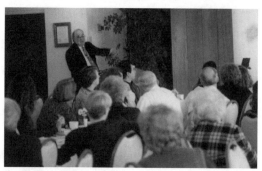ties in the form of lectures, conferences, newsletters, and books for the public as well as health care professionals.

The *RECNAC* cancer research project began in 1989. Its time limited goals are to discover by the year 2000 how and why cancer develops in humans, how to prevent it, and how to treat this dreaded disease using means which are not toxic to normal cells. The project is the major research thrust of the **Bio-Communications Research Institute**. The Institute also gathers clinical data about the effectiveness of the treatment protocols used by our doctors. *RECNAC* research is made possible by contributions from corporations, foundations, and hundreds of individuals.

The **Beat The Odds** program began as a pilot project in 1993. Designed for healthy people who want to stay that way, Beat The Odds provides the means for periodically monitoring the actual vitamin levels within individuals. This valuable program is especially appropriate for those with a family history of degenerative diseases such as Alzheimer's, arthritis, cancer, cataracts, diabetes, failing vision, heart disease, hypertension, or stroke. Beat The Odds is important for people taking nutrient supplements who want to know if they are absorbing and utilizing these nutrients.

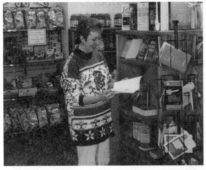

Other activities associated with The Center include the **Taste of Health** restaurant, the **Gift of Health** shop, the Luncheon Lecture series, and the **Delta Sigma Gamma** volunteer organization.

To learn more about The Center send a stamped self-addressed #10 envelope to:

The Center
3100 N. Hillside Avenue
Wichita, Kansas 67219 USA
316-682-3100

Visit our website at http://www.brightspot.org or come for a tour where you'll meet some of our staff.

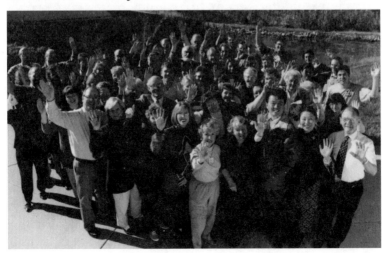

Special Offer

Now that you've learned the contents of *The Wonderful World Within You*, keep up-to-date wih the latest nutrition information by becoming a member of *HEALTH HUNTER*.

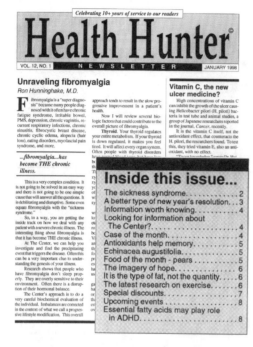

To get your own free issue of *Health Hunter*, just complete the coupon below and send with a stamped, self-addressed envelope to

Health Hunter
3100 North
Hillside Ave.
Wichita KS
67219 USA

or visit our website at http//www.brightspot.org.